The Steady
Ground Series

Talking to Young Children Ages 3–8

About Divorce & Parental Addiction

Answering the Hard Questions With Compassion and Clarity

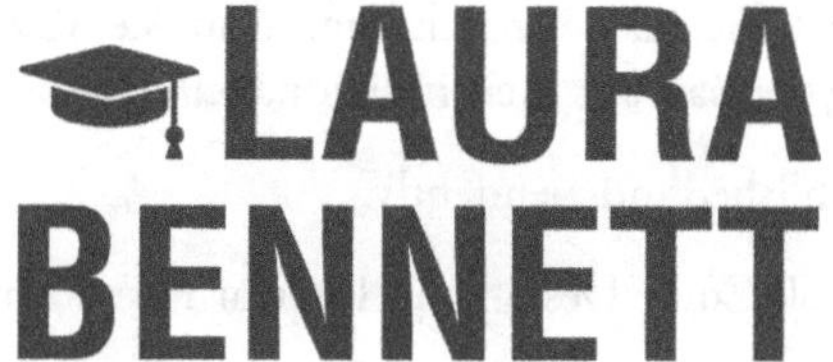

Published independently.

Book Cover Design and Interior Formatting by 100 Covers

ISBN: [Leave blank until assigned]

The Steady Ground Series

Guidance for Parents Supporting Young Children Ages 3–8 Through Change

The Steady Ground Series offers calm, developmentally informed guidance for parents navigating family change while raising young children. Each volume focuses on answering the hard questions children ask—or express through behavior—during times of disruption, using language that supports emotional safety, trust, and resilience.

These books are grounded in early childhood development and trauma-informed understanding. They are written for parents who want to respond with steadiness, clarity, and care—even when circumstances feel uncertain.

Children do not need perfect circumstances. They need at least one steady adult who understands what they are feeling.

Books in the Series

Talking to Young Children Ages 3–8 About Divorce and Parental Addiction: Answering the Hard Questions with Compassion and Clarity

Helping Young Children Ages 3–8 Navigate Life Between Two Homes: Answering the Hard Questions with Compassion and Clarity

How to Use This Book

This book is meant to be a steady presence—not something you rush through or try to apply all at once. You do not need to read it cover to cover in order. You may find yourself returning to certain sections as new questions arise or as your child's needs shift over time.

Some parents will read this book during the early days of separation. Others will return to it months later, when behaviors change or new questions surface. Both approaches are valid.

This book is not about doing divorce "right." It is about helping your child feel safe, loved, and anchored while life is changing.

TABLE OF CONTENTS

INTRODUCTION

Divorce is one of the most difficult decisions a parent will ever make. It arrives after sleepless nights, painful conversations, and the weight of knowing that life as a family once knew it will fundamentally change. For parents of young children, that weight is compounded by a question that echoes relentlessly: *What will this do to my child?*

This book was written for parents navigating that question—not with judgment, but with compassion and clarity. It speaks directly to those who lie awake at night, wondering if their three-year-old's sudden clinginess is normal, if their six-year-old's angry outbursts mean lasting damage, or if their eight-year-old's quiet withdrawal signals something they should have prevented. It is for parents who are trying to hold their children steady while their own world feels uncertain, who want to protect their child's emotional wellbeing even when adult circumstances are complicated and messy.

This book is part of the Answering the Hard Questions series, created to help parents respond to young children's fears and questions with honesty, steadiness, and care.

Here's what the research tells us, and it might surprise you: divorce itself doesn't determine a child's long-term emotional health—what matters most is how we as parents show up during and after the transition. What developmental psychologists have found is this: when children experience divorce alongside responsive, attuned parenting and consistent emotional support, they demonstrate resilience and healthy adjustment over time. What matters far more than the family structure itself is the quality of your relationship with your child, the stability of your routines, and your child's sense of safety.

Young children between the ages of three and eight experience divorce through a unique developmental lens. They lack the cognitive capacity to understand abstract concepts like "growing apart" or "incompatibility," and instead interpret family change through concrete, immediate questions: Where will I sleep? Will Mommy come back? Did I somehow make Daddy leave? Their emotional responses often show up through behavior rather than words—regression in toileting or sleep, increased tantrums, withdrawal from play, or heightened anxiety about separation. For children with neurodivergence or heightened sensory sensitivity, these responses may be intensified—transitions and unpredictability can be particularly challenging when developing nervous systems process emotions and sensory information differently.

This guide also addresses the real, difficult questions you face when divorce involves more than logistical changes. When one parent struggles with substance abuse, when shared parenting feels impossible because the other parent is uncooperative or emotionally volatile, when safety concerns mean supervised visits or limited contact—these situations require more than generic advice about amicable separation. You need guidance rooted in reality, not idealized scenarios that don't match your lived experience.

This book provides exactly that guidance. Throughout these chapters, you'll find practical, actionable strategies grounded in child development research and clinical expertise from psychologists who work with both typically developing children and neurodivergent children experiencing family disruption. The focus remains consistently on what children need to feel safe, loved, and anchored during change—and on empowering you to provide that foundation even when you're grieving, exhausted, or overwhelmed.

This book also offers something equally important: permission. Permission to have hard days, to prioritize self-care without guilt, and to set boundaries with an ex-partner when necessary. Permission to acknowledge that parenting through divorce is extraordinarily difficult, and that doing it imperfectly while remaining present and responsive is enough.

This matters because children are remarkably resilient when they feel seen, heard, and safe. You don't need to shield your children from all difficult emotions or maintain perfect composure at all times. Instead, what children need is a parent who notices their distress, responds with warmth and consistency, and helps them make sense of their changing world with honesty and reassurance. This book provides the tools, language, and understanding to do exactly that—one conversation, one moment of repair, one predictable routine at a time.

You'll see this message repeated throughout the book: this is not your fault. That repetition is intentional. Parents navigating divorce and addiction often carry layers of guilt that resurface in different moments. Repeating this reassurance isn't about convincing you once—it's about meeting you wherever you are when the doubt returns.

CHAPTER 1

What Your Child May Be Feeling Right Now

Understanding Divorce and Change Through Young Eyes

The decision to divorce is never made lightly, and if you're reading this, you've likely spent countless hours weighing what's best for yourself and your children. You may be carrying guilt, uncertainty, or fear about how this change will shape your young one's life—and that concern itself is a sign of your deep love and commitment to their wellbeing. What you're doing right now—seeking to understand your child's experience, looking for ways to support them through this transition—matters more than you might realize.

This chapter won't tell you that divorce is easy on children, because that wouldn't be true. But it will help you see the world through your young child's eyes so you can respond to what they actually need rather than what you fear they might be feeling.

Children between the ages of three and eight live in a different emotional reality than adults do. They don't understand divorce as a legal process or even as a relationship ending. They experience it as a disruption to everything that has made them feel safe: the predictability of who will be there when they wake up, the familiar sounds of both parents' voices in the home, the unquestioned certainty that their world will remain intact.

You may notice this idea appearing again throughout the book: young children communicate distress through behavior rather than words. This repetition is intentional. It's one of the most important concepts for understanding children during times of change.

When that foundation shifts, children don't have the cognitive tools to make sense of it the way older children or adults might. They can't yet think abstractly about concepts like "growing apart" or "what's best for the family." Instead, they interpret change through their bodies, their behaviors, and their immediate emotional responses.

This is why your four-year-old might suddenly refuse to sleep alone after months of independent bedtime, or why your seven-year-old who never had tantrums now melts down over seemingly small frustrations. These behaviors aren't manipulation or defiance—they're communication. Your child is showing you, in the only language available to them at this developmental stage, that their sense of safety has been shaken and they need help finding solid ground again.

For some children, this experience is even more intense. Children with neurodivergent profiles—those with autism, ADHD, dyslexia, or other differences in how they process the world—often rely heavily on routine, predictability, and clear expectations to manage daily life. When divorce disrupts these anchors, the distress can be profound and the behavioral responses more extreme. Children with heightened sensitivity, who experience emotions and sensory input more intensely than their peers, may seem overwhelmed by feelings they can't name or regulate. These children aren't being difficult; they're showing you how hard they're working to make sense of a world that suddenly feels unstable.

Understanding what your child is experiencing doesn't require you to have all the answers or to manage this transition perfectly. It doesn't mean you need to hide your own emotions or pretend everything is fine when it isn't. What it does require is a willingness to notice, to listen not just to words but to behavior, and to respond with compassion even when you're exhausted and uncertain yourself.

Throughout this chapter, you'll learn how young children perceive and process divorce differently at various developmental stages, what safety truly means from a child's perspective, and how to read the signals your child is sending through their behavior rather than their words. You'll gain insight into how neurodivergent and highly sensitive children may experience this transition with particular intensity, and what that means for how you support them.

This isn't about doing divorce "right." It's about helping your child feel anchored, loved, and safe even as their world changes—and trusting that your presence, your attention, and your willingness to see them clearly will make all the difference.

How Young Children Understand Change: The Developmental Reality of Divorce for Ages 3-8

Here's what's important to understand: young children between three and eight experience divorce completely differently depending on their age, and they simply can't grasp abstract ideas like relationship dissolution or what this might mean for their future. A three-year-old and an eight-year-old going through the same divorce will tell themselves completely different stories about what's happening and why—each making sense of it through the only lens available to them at that age.

To understand how young children process divorce, we need to start with how their brains actually work at this age. Three- and four-year-olds are in what developmental psychologists call the preoperational stage—which basically means they think concretely and see the world primarily from their own perspective. They cannot yet understand cause-and-effect relationships in complex situations, nor can they separate their own perspective from others' experiences.

When parents separate, preschoolers don't wonder about compatibility or adult emotional needs—they fixate on immediate, tangible concerns. Rhonda Freeman, who manages the Families in Transition program at Toronto's Family Services Association, explains that with their limited cognitive ability, three- and four-year-olds can develop inaccurate ideas about the causes and effects of divorce, often believing they somehow caused the separation or that a parent left them personally rather than the marriage.

This age group's questions reveal their developmental reality: "Where will the cat live?" "Who's going to look after me?" "Will I still have my bedroom?" These aren't trivial concerns—they represent a child's entire framework for understanding safety and continuity.

California psychologist and divorce researcher Joan B. Kelly notes that adults see divorce for the complex, multifaceted situation it is, while young children tend to view it in concrete and self-centered terms, meaning big-picture reassurances about ongoing parental love may mean little to a child wondering about their hamster's living arrangements.

Preschoolers also lack the temporal understanding to grasp concepts like "next weekend" or "in a few months." When a parent says they'll see the child soon, that child has no meaningful way to measure or anticipate that timeframe. This cognitive limitation intensifies separation anxiety and makes transitions between homes particularly distressing, as each goodbye can feel permanent to a three-year-old who cannot yet hold the concept of future reunion.

As children move into ages five through eight, their cognitive abilities expand significantly, though critical limitations remain. Early school-age children begin to understand that divorce is a word with meaning, that other families experience it too, and that their parents' separation involves some kind of conflict or incompatibility. They can ask more sophisticated questions and engage in longer conversations about what's happening, though their reasoning remains bound by what researchers call "fantastical reasoning" and concrete logic.

A kindergartener might conclude that divorce happened because Dad deleted something from Mom's computer—an actual question one Toronto parent received from her daughter—revealing the child's attempt to impose logical cause-and-effect on an incomprehensible adult situation. An eight-year-old might wonder if their bedtime misbehavior caused enough stress to break up the marriage. These aren't irrational fears from a child's perspective; they represent genuine attempts to understand using the cognitive tools available at that developmental stage.

Children in this age range also begin to care deeply about peer relationships and social context. They may worry about telling friends, wonder if divorce makes their family different or wrong, and struggle with questions about why this is happening to them. Even as they become more independent and seek stability through friendships and school routines, they still fundamentally depend on their parents' presence and predictability to manage their emotions.

Across all ages in this developmental window, children share one critical limitation: they cannot think abstractly about relationships, future possibilities, or emotional complexity the way adults can. They experience divorce not as a concept but as a series of concrete disruptions to the physical and emotional landscape that has always defined safety. Understanding this developmental reality allows parents to meet children where they actually are rather than where adults wish they could be.

What Safety Means to a Young Child: Attachment, Routine, and Predictability During Transition

To understand how divorce disrupts a child's world, we must first understand what safety means to them. Safety, for a young child, is not an abstract concept they can articulate or even fully recognize. It exists in the felt experience of their daily life—in the predictable rhythm of morning routines, in the certainty that a trusted adult will be there at pickup time, in the familiar sound of a parent's voice reading the same bedtime story night after night. When divorce disrupts these patterns, children don't think "my sense of security has been compromised." They simply feel unmoored, anxious, and uncertain in ways their developing brains struggle to process or communicate.

Here's what attachment research shows us: children's sense of safety is fundamentally rooted in their relationships with primary caregivers. Psychologist

John Bowlby's foundational work showed us that children develop secure emotional bonds when they experience consistent, responsive care from at least one reliable adult. This secure base allows children to explore their world, regulate their emotions, and develop healthy relationships throughout life. During divorce, this attachment system is activated intensely because the child's brain perceives a threat to the very foundation of their survival—the stability of their caregiving relationships.

For children ages three through eight, attachment manifests in concrete, observable ways. A securely attached four-year-old knows that when they fall and scrape their knee, their parent will respond with comfort. They trust that bedtime will follow a familiar sequence, that meals will appear at expected times, and that the adults in their life will be emotionally available when needed—certainties that divorce threatens simultaneously, even when parents are doing their best to maintain stability.

The disruption is particularly acute because young children lack the cognitive capacity to understand that their parent's physical absence from the home doesn't mean abandonment or loss of love. A six-year-old whose father now lives in a different house may experience genuine grief and fear each time that parent leaves after a visit, unable to hold the abstract concept that "Dad still loves me even though he doesn't live here anymore." The child's attachment system registers only the concrete reality: the person I depend on is leaving, and I don't know when they'll return.

Routine provides the scaffolding that supports attachment security during periods of transition. Child development researchers have consistently found that predictable daily patterns help regulate children's nervous systems, reducing cortisol levels and allowing the brain's executive functioning to develop properly. When a child knows what to expect—that breakfast happens before getting dressed, that Wednesday is always a day with Mom, that Saturday mornings mean pancakes with Dad—their cognitive resources can focus on learning and growth rather than hypervigilance and anxiety.

Divorce inevitably disrupts routine, even in the most amicable separations. The child who once woke up in the same bed every morning now alternates between two homes. Mealtimes may differ between households. One parent may have different rules about screen time or bedtime. For neurotypical children, these changes require significant adjustment. For children with neurodivergent profiles—particularly those with autism or ADHD who rely heavily on routine for emotion regulation—the loss of predictability can be profoundly destabilizing, sometimes triggering developmental regression or intensified anxiety that parents struggle to understand.

Predictability extends beyond daily schedules to include emotional consistency. Young children need to know not just where they'll be and when, but also that the adults caring for them will respond in relatively consistent ways. A child who cannot predict whether their parent will be patient or irritable, present or distracted, available or overwhelmed, experiences this inconsistency as a form of emotional unsafety. This doesn't mean parents must be perfect or never show difficult emotions—it means that children need to experience their parents as fundamentally reliable in their responsiveness and care, even when circumstances are hard.

The work of maintaining safety during divorce transition, then, centers on preserving as much attachment security, routine, and predictability as possible while acknowledging that some disruption is inevitable. Parents cannot prevent all change, but they can be intentional about which anchors they protect and how they help their children navigate the shifts that must occur.

Reading the Signals: How Children Communicate Distress Through Behavior Rather Than Words

Understanding what safety means to children naturally leads to the question of how they communicate when that safety feels threatened. When a child cannot find words for what they're feeling, their body and behavior become the messenger.

A seven-year-old who suddenly refuses to get dressed for school isn't being defiant—they may be showing you that the transition between homes has become overwhelming. A five-year-old who has started wetting the bed after months of being dry isn't regressing out of laziness—they're communicating that their sense of security has been shaken in ways they cannot articulate.

For young children navigating divorce, behavior is language, and learning to read these signals is one of the most important skills a parent can develop during this transition.

Here's what research in child development consistently shows: children ages three through eight lack both the emotional vocabulary and the cognitive capacity to directly express complex feelings about family disruption.

Instead, distress manifests through observable changes in daily functioning, emotion regulation, and social behavior. Clinical psychologist and divorce researcher Joan Kelly points out that behavioral changes serve as critical indicators of a child's internal experience, particularly when those changes represent departures from the child's typical patterns.

Separation anxiety and clinginess often intensify dramatically during divorce, even in children who previously separated easily from parents. A four-year-old who once happily went to preschool may now cling to a parent's leg at drop-off, crying inconsolably. This behavior reflects the child's fear that when a parent leaves, they might not return—a reasonable concern from a developmental perspective when one parent has already left the family home. The child's attachment system has been activated by perceived threat, and proximity-seeking behavior is the brain's attempt to restore safety.

Behavioral regressions represent another common signal of distress. Children may lose skills they had previously mastered—toilet training, independent sleeping, self-feeding, or age-appropriate speech. A six-year-old might suddenly ask for a bottle or speak in baby talk. These regressions aren't manipulation; they're the nervous system's response to overwhelming stress.

When a child uses all their emotional energy trying to make sense of family changes, they have less capacity left for maintaining skills that require ongoing effort and self-regulation. As one expert notes, "Behavioral regressions, such as bedwetting or thumb-sucking, [occur] as young children try to cope with the changes."

Aggression and acting out frequently emerge as outlets for feelings children cannot name or process verbally. A typically gentle eight-year-old might suddenly hit classmates, destroy toys, or explode in rage over minor frustrations. Child psychologists recognize this behavior as externalized distress—the child is showing rather than telling that they're carrying anger, confusion, or fear about circumstances beyond their control.

In high-conflict divorces where children witness parental arguments, aggression often intensifies as children absorb and mirror the emotional volatility they're exposed to. As research confirms, "Children often act out in response to the emotional turmoil of divorce. Behavioral problems such as aggression, irritability, or defiance can arise, particularly in children who have difficulty expressing their emotions verbally."

Conversely, some children respond to divorce-related distress through **withdrawal and emotional shutdown.** A previously social seven-year-old might stop engaging with friends, lose interest in activities they once loved, or spend hours in solitary, repetitive play. This withdrawal signals that the child feels emotionally overwhelmed and is attempting to protect themselves by reducing stimulation and interaction.

Clinical observations indicate that withdrawal can be particularly concerning because it's quieter and less disruptive than acting out, sometimes causing parents to miss the depth of the child's struggle. Child counseling perspectives note:

"Indicators that your child may be having difficulties coping... [include] behavioral problems like attention seeking, 'acting out', mood swings or prolonged sadness/ depression, apathy or loss of interest."

Changes in sleep and eating patterns also communicate distress nonverbally. Nightmares, bedtime resistance, middle-of-the-night waking, or requests to co-sleep all reflect heightened anxiety and disrupted feelings of safety. Similarly, appetite changes—whether refusing food or seeking constant snacks—can indicate that the child's stress response system is dysregulated.

For children with neurodivergent profiles, these behavioral signals may be amplified or expressed differently. A child with autism might show increased stimming behaviors, sensory sensitivities, or rigid adherence to routines as ways of managing the additional stress divorce brings to their already-demanding work of navigating daily life. A child with ADHD might display intensified impulsivity, emotional outbursts, or difficulty focusing as their executive functioning resources become overtaxed.

Understanding that behavior is communication allows parents to respond with curiosity rather than frustration, asking not "Why are you acting this way?" but rather "What are you trying to tell me?"

The Intensified Experience: Understanding Divorce Through the Lens of Neurodivergence and High Sensitivity

While all young children struggle to communicate distress through behavior, some children face additional challenges that intensify their experience. For some children, the experience of divorce isn't simply difficult—it's overwhelming in ways that exceed what their nervous systems can manage without significant support.

Children with neurodivergent profiles and those who are highly sensitive experience family transitions with an intensity that can surprise even well-prepared parents. These children aren't being dramatic or manipulative. Their neurological differences mean they genuinely process change, emotion, and sensory input differently than their neurotypical peers, and divorce activates these differences in profound ways.

Children with neurodivergent profiles—including those with autism spectrum disorder, ADHD, sensory processing variations, or learning disabilities—often rely heavily on routine, predictability, and clear expectations to navigate daily life successfully.

In an interview featured on The Autism Dad, psychologist Dr. Mikki Lee emphasized that consistency forms the foundation of emotional regulation and security for many neurodivergent children (Gorski, 2025). When divorce disrupts routines that have scaffolded a child's world, the impact can be destabilizing in ways that extend beyond typical adjustment challenges.

A six-year-old with autism who has always followed the same morning sequence—wake up, find Dad making coffee in the kitchen, eat the same breakfast at the same table, follow the same getting-ready routine—may experience genuine distress when Dad no longer lives in the home.

This isn't resistance to change or an inability to be flexible; it's a neurological reality—the child's brain has organized itself around these patterns, using them to predict what comes next and to manage the sensory and emotional demands of each day. When those patterns dissolve, the child loses critical tools for regulation, often resulting in behaviors that look like regression, defiance, or emotional meltdown but are actually communication about overwhelm.

Children with ADHD face different but equally significant challenges during divorce. Executive function—the brain's ability to plan, organize, manage emotions, and shift between tasks—is already an area of struggle for children with ADHD. Divorce introduces multiple additional demands on executive function simultaneously: adapting to two different homes with different rules, remembering which belongings go where, managing transitions between parents, and processing complex emotions about family change.

For a seven-year-old whose executive function is already overtaxed by ordinary daily demands, these additional requirements can result in increased impulsivity, emotional outbursts, difficulty focusing at school, and what appears to be oppositional behavior but is actually cognitive overload.

Children with heightened sensitivity, whether neurodivergent or neurotypical, experience emotions and sensory input more intensely than their peers. Developmental psychologist Elaine Aron's research has shown that approximately fifteen to twenty percent of children are born with a more sensitive nervous system, processing stimuli more deeply and reacting more strongly to emotional environments.

During divorce, these children may become hyperaware of parental tension, picking up on subtle shifts in mood or tone that other children might miss. They may feel their own emotions about the divorce with such intensity that they struggle to function—unable to sleep because worry feels physically overwhelming, unable to eat because anxiety sits heavy in their stomach, unable to concentrate at school because their mind is consumed with fears they cannot articulate.

For all of these children, the abstract nature of divorce concepts creates additional confusion. A four-year-old with autism may not understand what "Mommy and Daddy don't live together anymore" actually means in concrete terms.

Without visual supports and explicit, repeated explanations, the child may develop their own narrative—one that often centers on self-blame or catastrophic fears. Sara Olsher, who navigated divorce while parenting her neurodivergent daughter, discovered that children invent stories when adults don't provide clear information, and those invented stories almost always place the child at the center of blame.

Understanding these intensified experiences allows parents to respond with appropriate support rather than frustration when their neurodivergent or highly sensitive child struggles more visibly than siblings or peers during the divorce transition.

The journey through divorce with young children doesn't require you to have perfect answers or to shield your child from all difficult emotions. What it requires is something you're already doing by reading these words: a willingness to see your child's experience clearly, to understand that their reality differs fundamentally from your own, and to respond with intention rather than assumption.

The developmental lens through which children ages three through eight perceive divorce—concrete, egocentric, rooted in immediate sensory and emotional experience rather than abstract understanding—shapes everything about how they process this transition and what they need from you as they navigate it.

Your child's behavior in the coming weeks and months will tell you stories their words cannot. The clinginess, the regressions, the sudden tantrums or quiet withdrawal—these aren't signs that you've damaged your child irreparably or that divorce was the wrong choice. They're communication from a developing nervous system working hard to make sense of profound change with limited cognitive tools and immature emotion regulation capacities.

Responding to these behaviors with curiosity rather than frustration, with reassurance rather than dismissal, teaches your child something essential: that their feelings matter, that they're not alone in their confusion or fear, and that you remain a steady presence even when their world feels uncertain.

For parents of neurodivergent or children with heightened sensitivity, this work may feel more demanding because the signals are often more intense and the need for routine and predictability more acute.

These children aren't being difficult—they're showing you how much harder their nervous systems have to work to manage transitions that already challenge neurotypical children. Understanding this difference allows you to offer support that matches your child's actual needs rather than comparing their adjustment to developmental expectations that don't account for neurodivergence.

The foundation of safety you're building now—through maintained routines where possible, through consistent emotional presence, through your willingness to repair connection after hard moments—matters more than any single conversation or perfect explanation ever could.

Research in attachment and child development consistently demonstrates that children are remarkably resilient when they have at least one reliable, responsive adult who helps them make sense of their experience and who remains emotionally available even amid stress and change. You are that person for your child, and your commitment to understanding their inner world is already providing the anchor they need.

As you move forward through this book, you'll gain specific language for talking with your child about divorce, concrete strategies for managing difficult behaviors and big emotions, and practical tools for maintaining your own wellbeing while supporting theirs.

You'll learn how to navigate complicated situations—when the other parent is struggling with addiction, when visits don't go as planned, when your child's feelings about both parents become confusing and contradictory. But all of these specific skills rest on the foundation established in this chapter: the recognition that your child's experience of divorce is fundamentally different from yours, that behavior is their primary language for distress, and that your attuned, responsive presence is the most powerful tool you have for helping them feel safe.

You don't need to eliminate your child's difficult feelings or prevent all behavioral struggles. You need to help them feel accompanied through the hard moments, to know that their confusion and fear make sense, and to trust that the ground beneath them—your love, your presence, your commitment to their wellbeing—remains solid even when so much else has changed.

That work begins not with perfect words or flawless execution, but with exactly what you're doing now: paying attention, seeking to understand, and showing up with compassion for both your child and yourself.

CHAPTER 2

When a Parent Is Struggling in Ways Children Can Sense

Talking Gently About Addiction Without Fear or Blame

Some of what you'll read in this chapter may sound familiar. That's intentional. When children are under stress, they need the same messages repeated in steady, predictable ways—and so do parents. Each time we return to these ideas, we're not circling back because nothing has changed, but because repetition helps build understanding, safety, and confidence over time.

When a parent struggles with addiction, the other parent often carries a weight that feels impossible to describe—the need to protect your child while watching someone you once trusted become unpredictable, the guilt of limiting contact, the exhaustion of being the steady one. You may wonder how much your child already knows, what you should say, and whether speaking the truth will cause more harm than silence.

The reality is that children are highly perceptive. Even very young children observe when a parent's behavior changes, when promises are broken repeatedly, when the adult who is supposed to care for them seems somehow absent even when physically present. They pick up on tension in your voice when you talk about the other parent, on the worry that tightens your shoulders when drop-off time approaches, and on the careful way you phrase explanations that don't quite explain anything.

Your three-year-old may not understand the word "addiction," but she knows that Daddy acts differently sometimes, that his hugs smell strange, and that he fell asleep during her birthday party.

Your seven-year-old may not grasp the neurobiology of addiction, but he knows that Mom promised to come to his soccer game and didn't, again, and that when she did show up last time, something felt wrong in a way he can't name.

Silence in the face of what children already sense doesn't protect them—it isolates them. When children observe troubling patterns but receive no explanation, they create their own stories to make sense of what they're experiencing.

These stories almost always center on the child's own responsibility: *Daddy wouldn't drink so much if I were better behaved. Mom cancels visits because I'm not lovable enough. If I were different, everything would be okay.* The absence of truthful, age-appropriate information leaves children alone with their observations, their fears, and their self-blame.

This chapter offers guidance for one of the hardest conversations you may ever have with your child: talking about a parent's struggle with addiction in ways that are honest without being frightening, that acknowledge reality without creating shame, and that help your child understand that addiction is an illness affecting someone they love—not a reflection of the child's worth or a burden the child must carry.

You'll find language that fits different developmental stages, strategies for answering the difficult questions that follow initial conversations, and support for navigating the ongoing challenge of helping your child maintain connection with a struggling parent when it's safe while setting necessary boundaries when it's not.

This chapter also acknowledges the particular pain you carry as the parent trying to create stability while the other parent's addiction creates chaos. Anger at your ex-partner for putting your child through this may consume you at times.

Grief follows—for the family you hoped to have, the co-parent you thought would show up, the relationship you wanted your child to have with both parents.

Guilt about necessary decisions (limiting visitation, documenting concerning behavior, involving courts or child protective services) weighs heavily, and you may wonder constantly whether you're protecting enough or inadvertently damaging your child's relationship with their other parent through honesty.

What follows is not about vilifying a struggling parent or eliminating a child's relationship with them. It's about helping you find words that tell the truth with compassion, that protect your child's emotional wellbeing while honoring their love for both parents, and that free your child from the impossible responsibility of fixing or explaining an adult's illness.

Your child deserves honesty that creates understanding rather than fear, and you deserve support for carrying the weight of being the parent who shows up, day after day, to provide the safety and consistency your child needs.

What Children Already Sense: Recognizing That Silence Doesn't Equal Protection

Young children possess what developmental psychologists describe as an extraordinary capacity for emotional attunement—they read facial expressions, body language, vocal tone, and environmental tension with remarkable accuracy, often detecting distress in caregivers before adults consciously recognize it themselves.

Research in attachment theory demonstrates that children as young as three years old monitor their parents' emotional states as a survival mechanism, constantly scanning for signs that their primary attachment figures are safe, available, and responsive.

When a parent struggles with addiction, children observe the inconsistencies, the mood shifts, the broken promises, and the subtle ways their parent seems different or unavailable, even when no one has spoken a word about what's happening.

Children naturally try to make sense of what they observe. As Tina Payne Bryson and Daniel Siegel explain, when adults do not provide clear, age-appropriate information, children often create their own explanations—and those explanations frequently center on self-blame (Bryson & Siegel, 2011).

A four-year-old who notices that Mommy sleeps through afternoon pickup and smells strange when she finally wakes up doesn't think, "My mother has a disease that affects her brain and behavior." Instead, that child thinks, "Mommy doesn't want to see me. I must have done something wrong. Maybe if I'm quieter, better, more helpful, she'll be okay."

This tendency toward self-blame is rooted in what developmental psychologist Jean Piaget identified as the egocentrism of early childhood—the cognitive limitation that makes young children believe they are the center of causation in their world.

Children in the early childhood developmental stage, roughly ages two through seven, struggle to understand that events can have causes unrelated to their own actions or worth. When they sense something is wrong and receive no explanation that counters this egocentric thinking, they default to the belief that they caused the problem or that something is fundamentally wrong with them.

The protective silence many parents choose—motivated by love and the desire to shield children from painful realities—actually amplifies children's distress rather than reducing it.

Drawing on trauma research, Bruce Perry's work highlights how unpredictable or frightening caregiver behavior can disrupt a child's developing nervous system and sense of safety (Greig et al., 2023).

When children observe that a parent is behaving unpredictably, that visits are frequently cancelled, that the other parent seems worried or angry when discussing their co-parent, but no one acknowledges these observations, children experience what researchers call "cognitive dissonance"—the psychological stress of holding two conflicting realities simultaneously.

They know something is wrong because they can see and feel it, yet the adults around them act as though everything is fine.

This dissonance is particularly acute for neurodivergent children, who may process social cues and uncertainty differently. Many autistic children benefit from predictability and clear, concrete information to feel safe.

When patterns change without explanation—a parent who was previously reliable becomes inconsistent, routines shift without warning—neurodivergent children may experience heightened anxiety and dysregulation.

Similarly, children with ADHD, who may experience managing emotions differently, can become overwhelmed by the unexplained tension they sense, leading to increased behavioral responses that parents may misinterpret as defiance rather than distress.

The research is clear: children benefit from age-appropriate honesty that validates what they're already sensing. Silence doesn't protect children from painful realities they've already observed—it only ensures they face those realities alone, without the reassurance, context, and support that truthful, compassionate communication provides.

Finding Words That Fit: Age-Appropriate Ways to Explain Addiction Without Creating Fear or Blame

Finding the right words to explain addiction to a young child requires balancing honesty with emotional safety, providing enough information to counter self-blame while avoiding details that create fear or overwhelm. The language parents choose matters deeply—not because there's one perfect script, but because children need explanations that match their developmental capacity to understand while validating what they've already observed.

For children ages three to five, explanations work best when they are concrete, brief, and connected to concepts the child already understands. As Tina Payne Bryson and Daniel Siegel explain, preschool-aged children tend to think in literal terms and may struggle with abstract concepts, making familiar comparisons especially helpful (Bryson & Siegel, 2011).

A parent might say: "You know how when you have a cold, your body doesn't feel right and you need medicine to get better? Daddy's brain has a sickness that makes him need alcohol to feel okay, even though the alcohol actually makes the sickness worse. It's not something you caused, and it's not something you can fix. Doctors and other helpers are the ones who can help him get better."

This explanation accomplishes several critical goals simultaneously. It names what the child has likely already noticed—that something is wrong with the parent.

It frames addiction as an illness rather than a moral failing or a choice the parent is making to hurt the child. It explicitly removes responsibility from the child.

And it identifies that adults, not children, are responsible for addressing the problem.

Children ages six to eight can handle slightly more nuanced explanations that acknowledge the brain science of addiction without overwhelming them with medical terminology. Research in developmental psychology shows that early elementary-aged children are beginning to understand cause and effect more clearly and can grasp that the same person can have both good qualities and struggles.

A parent might explain: "Mom's brain got used to needing drugs to feel normal, kind of like how your body gets used to eating at certain times and you feel really hungry if you don't eat. But drugs change how the brain works, and now her brain tells her she needs the drugs even though they're hurting her. She loves you very much, and the part of her that's sick is not the part that loves you. The sickness makes it hard for her to make good choices sometimes, but that's because of the addiction, not because of anything you did."

What parents should carefully avoid is language that vilifies the struggling parent, creates terror about substances, or suggests the child should feel responsible for monitoring or managing the parent's behavior.

Phrases like "Your father is a drunk" or "Mom cares more about drugs than about you" place the child in an impossible loyalty conflict and increase shame rather than understanding. Similarly, fear-based warnings—"If you ever try drugs, you'll become an addict just like your dad"—can create anxiety without providing useful information.

Bruce Perry's research reminds us that reassurance of safety can help children absorb difficult information more gently. After explaining addiction, caregivers can offer simple, comforting language such as:

"I know this can feel confusing. You are safe with me. I'm taking care of what you need, and there are people helping our family. You can always ask questions, and we will talk through them together."

For neurodivergent children who may need more concrete language and repetition, visual supports can help.

A simple drawing showing "Daddy's brain" with a note that "this part is sick and needs help" gives children something tangible to reference. Children with autism particularly benefit from clear, consistent language repeated across multiple conversations rather than one lengthy explanation.

The goal is not to explain addiction comprehensively in one conversation, but to open a dialogue that continues as the child grows and new questions emerge.

Balancing Love and Safety: Navigating Contact, Boundaries, and the Child's Relationship with a Struggling Parent

One of the most painful realities parents face when a co-parent struggles with addiction is the tension between wanting to preserve the child's relationship with that parent and needing to protect the child from harm.

Children ages three to eight are developmentally wired to love both parents, regardless of those parents' struggles or limitations. Attachment research demonstrates that children maintain deep emotional bonds with caregivers even when those caregivers are inconsistent, unreliable, or sometimes frightening—a phenomenon attachment theorists call "insecure attachment."

The child's love for a struggling parent is real, powerful, and not something that should be dismissed or discouraged, even when that parent's behavior creates legitimate safety concerns.

When navigating contact and caregiving decisions, gently prioritizing a child's emotional and physical sense of safety can provide important stability. Bruce Perry's trauma research highlights that children who experience unpredictability or fear in caregiving relationships may find it harder to feel secure, which can influence their developing capacity for trust and emotional regulation.

When a parent is actively using substances, their behavior becomes unpredictable in ways that young children find terrifying—the parent who seems loving one moment may become angry, sleepy, or emotionally absent the next, leaving children confused about whether they are safe and whether the parent they love is still present.

The challenge, then, is creating boundaries that protect children while honoring their need for connection. This doesn't mean eliminating contact entirely in most situations, but rather structuring contact in ways that minimize risk while maximizing the child's sense of safety and predictability.

Family courts and child welfare professionals often recommend supervised visitation when a parent's addiction creates safety concerns—visits that occur in the presence of a neutral third party, whether a professional supervisor, a trusted family member, or in a designated visitation center. Supervised visits allow children to maintain their relationship with the struggling parent while ensuring that an adult is present to intervene if the parent's behavior becomes concerning.

For very young children, particularly those ages three to five, shorter, more frequent visits often work better than longer, less frequent contact.

Preschool-aged children have limited capacity to hold a parent in mind when that parent is absent, and extended separations can feel like abandonment.

Brief, consistent visits—even if supervised and limited to an hour or two — help maintain the relationship without overwhelming the child or exposing them to extended periods of potential unpredictability.

Parents managing these arrangements should communicate boundaries to children in language that emphasizes safety without vilifying the other parent.

Instead of saying, "You can't be alone with Daddy because he drinks too much and might hurt you," a parent might say, "Right now, visits with Daddy happen at the visit center where there are helpers to make sure everyone is safe and has a good time. Daddy loves you, and I love you, and we're all working to make sure you feel safe."

This language accomplishes several goals: it acknowledges the reality of changed circumstances, it reassures the child of both parents' love, and it frames the boundary as protective rather than punitive.

Changes in visits often bring questions, as children try to understand what is different and why. Tina Payne Bryson encourages caregivers to respond with calm, honest explanations that fit the child's developmental level, helping children feel supported rather than left to fill in the gaps on their own (Bryson & Siegel, 2011).

A parent might respond: "Mommy's sickness makes it hard for her to take care of you safely right now, so we're making sure visits happen in places where other grown-ups can help. When her sickness gets better, things might change. But right now, this is what keeps you safe."

Throughout these conversations and transitions, children need repeated reassurance that the boundaries are not their fault, that both parents love them, and that the adults are handling the grown-up problems.

Holding Space for Complicated Feelings: Helping Children Process Confusion, Anger, Worry, and Grief

When a parent struggles with addiction, children experience a particularly complex constellation of emotions that often exist simultaneously and contradict one another.

A six-year-old may feel angry that Mom missed her school play, worried that something bad will happen to Mom, confused about why Mom acts so differently sometimes, and grief-stricken over the loss of the parent she remembers from before—all within the same afternoon.

These feelings don't arrive neatly, one at a time, waiting to be processed and resolved before the next appears. They layer and shift, sometimes colliding in ways that leave children overwhelmed and parents uncertain how to help.

Research in developmental psychology demonstrates that children ages three to eight lack the cognitive capacity and emotional vocabulary to identify and articulate complex feelings without adult support.

Dan Siegel's research highlights that young children often feel emotions in their bodies and through their behavior long before language can capture those experiences. Worry may look like extra closeness, and big feelings such as anger or sadness can spill out during moments of frustration. These reactions reflect real emotional experiences, even when children do not yet have the words or understanding to share them directly.

Holding space for these complicated feelings means creating an environment where children can experience their emotions without judgment, without being rushed to "feel better," and without the burden of protecting adults from their pain.

It requires parents to resist the natural urge to fix, minimize, or redirect difficult emotions and instead to sit with children in their confusion, validate their anger, acknowledge their worry, and witness their grief.

Tina Payne Bryson emphasizes that validation is simply the process of helping children feel seen and understood. It does not mean agreeing with every interpretation or allowing all behavior, but instead communicating that their feelings are real and worthy of care while they continue learning healthier ways to respond (Bryson & Siegel, 2011).

When a seven-year-old says, "I hate Daddy for missing my birthday again," the validating response isn't "You don't really hate him" or "He couldn't help it because he's sick."

Instead, it's "You're really angry and hurt that he wasn't there. Birthdays are important, and you wanted him to be part of yours. It makes sense that you feel mad about that."

This response acknowledges the child's reality without requiring them to suppress legitimate anger or prematurely forgive.

For younger children who lack the language to express feelings verbally, parents can offer words that match what they observe in the child's behavior and body language. "I notice your body seems really tense and your voice sounds angry. I wonder if you're feeling frustrated about something" gives a four-year-old a starting point for connecting internal experience with external expression.

Over time and with repeated practice, children internalize this process and begin to develop their own capacity for emotional awareness.

Confusion often manifests as repetitive questioning—children ask the same questions about the divorce, about the other parent's behavior, about what will happen next, not because they didn't hear or understand the answer, but because they're trying to make sense of something that feels senseless.

Trauma research, including Bruce Perry's work, reminds us that young children often rely on repetition as they try to process experiences that feel confusing or overwhelming. Repeated questions—like "Why can't Mommy stop drinking?"—are less about testing patience and more about a child's attempt to make sense of something that does not match their understanding of how parents are supposed to behave.

Grief in young children often looks different than adult grief, manifesting in ways that can surprise or confuse parents. Children may seem fine one moment and devastated the next. They may play happily and then suddenly dissolve into tears, but this isn't emotional instability—it's developmentally normal grief processing.

Young children move in and out of painful feelings because they cannot sustain intense emotion for extended periods, needing breaks from their grief that often take the form of play—which simultaneously serves as respite and becomes a vehicle for processing loss through symbolic reenactment.

Talking to young children about a parent's addiction is one of the most difficult conversations a parent will ever navigate, and there is no script that makes it easy or painless. What research and clinical experience consistently demonstrate, however, is that children benefit profoundly from age-appropriate honesty that validates what they've already sensed, removes the burden of self-blame, and provides reassurance about their safety and their right to love both parents.

The silence that feels protective actually isolates children with their observations and fears, while truthful, compassionate communication—even when it acknowledges painful realities—helps children feel less alone and more anchored during uncertainty.

The language parents choose matters, not because there's one perfect way to explain addiction, but because children need explanations that match their developmental capacity while countering the egocentric thinking that leads them to believe they caused or can fix a parent's struggle.

Framing addiction as an illness that affects the brain helps young children understand that their parent's behavior isn't a reflection of the child's worth or a choice the parent is making to hurt them. Explicitly stating "This is not your fault, and you cannot fix it" directly addresses the self-blame that children carry when left to make sense of addiction on their own.

Balancing a child's need for connection with their need for safety requires difficult decisions that many parents face alone. Supervised visitation, modified custody arrangements, and clear boundaries around contact are not acts of punishment or alienation—they are protective measures that allow children to maintain relationships with struggling parents while minimizing exposure to unpredictable or frightening behavior.

Children can simultaneously love a parent deeply and need protection from that parent's illness, and holding both truths is part of the complex reality of parenting through a co-parent's addiction.

The emotions children experience in these circumstances—confusion, anger, worry, grief, and love all tangled together—don't resolve quickly or neatly. Children need ongoing permission to feel contradictory things at the same time, to be angry at a parent they also miss, to worry about someone whose choices have hurt them.

Parents who can sit with these complicated feelings without rushing to fix them, minimize them, or redirect them give children the invaluable gift of emotional companionship. Validation doesn't mean agreeing with every interpretation or endorsing harmful behavior—it means communicating that the child's feelings make sense given what they're experiencing, and that they don't have to carry those feelings alone.

For parents managing the weight of being the steady one while watching a co-parent struggle, the exhaustion and grief are real. The anger at broken promises, the fear during transitions, the guilt about limiting contact, the loneliness of making hard decisions without support—these feelings deserve acknowledgment too.

Protecting a child from a parent's addiction is not the same as keeping a child from a parent they love. It's creating the conditions under which love can exist safely, where the child's wellbeing is prioritized even when that requires boundaries the struggling parent may not understand or accept.

The conversations begun in this chapter are not one-time events but ongoing dialogues that will evolve as children grow, as circumstances change, and as new questions emerge. What remains constant is the child's need for honesty paired with reassurance, for information that creates understanding rather than fear, and for the presence of at least one parent who shows up consistently to provide safety, validation, and the unwavering message: *You are loved. This is not your fault. You are not alone.*

CHAPTER 3

Big Feelings in Little Hearts

Fear, Anger, Confusion, and the Need to Feel Safe

You might recognize some of the words used in this chapter. The reason we keep coming back to these concepts is not because nothing has changed; rather, it is because doing so gradually fosters comprehension, security, and self-assurance. That was deliberate. Both parents and children benefit from hearing the same soothing words expressed in consistent, predictable ways when times are tough.

Your five-year-old who once happily went to preschool now clings to your leg each morning, tears streaming, begging you not to leave. Your seven-year-old, typically gentle and cooperative, suddenly erupts in rage over small frustrations—a broken crayon, the wrong color cup—screaming words that shock you both.

These moments can feel bewildering and frightening, especially when you're already carrying the weight of managing a separation or divorce. You may find yourself wondering if you've broken something fundamental in your child, if these big reactions mean lasting damage, or if you're somehow failing to provide what they need.

The truth is both simpler and more complex: your child is communicating the only way they know how right now, and what they're saying is "I don't feel safe, and I need help making sense of what's happening."

Young children between the ages of three and eight are navigating divorce during a developmental window when their emotional regulation skills are still forming, their understanding of cause and effect remains limited, and their entire sense of security rests on the stability of their attachment relationships.

When that foundation shifts—when parents separate, when routines change, when one parent struggles with addiction or becomes less available—kids face a threat to their core sense of safety that they cannot yet name or understand.

Instead, that threat emerges as fear, anger, confusion, and an urgent, sometimes desperate need for reassurance.

This chapter explores these four primary emotional responses and what drives them from your child's developmental perspective.

Fear in young children during divorce isn't abstract worry about the future — it's an immediate, body-level response to perceived threats to attachment and predictability.

Anger often surprises parents with its intensity, but it serves as a young child's way of protesting powerlessness and attempting to regain some control in a world that suddenly feels chaotic.

Confusion stems not from a lack of explanation but from cognitive limitations that make abstract concepts like "divorce" nearly impossible for young minds to grasp, leaving children to fill in gaps with their own frightening interpretations.

And beneath all of these emotions lies the fundamental need to feel safe—not just physically protected, but emotionally held and relationally secure.

For children with neurodevelopmental differences and those who are highly sensitive, these emotional experiences often arrive with amplified intensity.

A child with autism may show distress through increased rigidity, meltdowns over minor changes, or withdrawal into repetitive behaviors.

A child with ADHD may become more impulsive, hyperactive, or emotionally explosive as their already-challenged regulation systems become further taxed.

Children with sensory sensitivities may experience physical symptoms—stomachaches, headaches, sleep disruptions—as their bodies respond to emotional overwhelm they cannot yet process verbally.

You don't need to eliminate these big feelings or prevent your child from experiencing any distress. That's neither possible nor necessary.

What matters is that you learn to recognize what your child is communicating through their behavior, that you respond with presence and validation rather than dismissal or punishment, and that you build consistent practices for helping them feel anchored even when life feels uncertain.

This chapter will help you understand what's happening beneath the surface when your child's emotions feel too big for their small body, and it will offer you practical, compassionate strategies for responding in ways that build safety rather than shame.

Your child's big feelings are not evidence of your failure—they're invitations for connection, and you have the capacity to answer them with the steadiness they need.

Fear and Anxiety in Young Children: Understanding Separation Distress, Regression, and the Threat to Attachment Security

Fear in young children during divorce operates at a primal level, rooted in the biological imperative for proximity to caregivers.

When family structure fractures, children face what attachment researchers identify as a threat to their primary survival system—the bond with parents that has kept humans alive for millennia.

I know this might sound dramatic, but it genuinely reflects the neurological reality of how young brains process separation and change. This concept will come up repeatedly while discussing cognitive developmental reactions. It is not because circumstances have changed, but because this is how you should understand your child's behavior.

Separation distress emerges when children perceive threats to their attachment security, whether through physical separation, emotional unavailability, or unpredictable parenting. During divorce, these threats multiply rapidly.

A parent who once reliably tucked them in at night now lives elsewhere. The other parent, overwhelmed by stress or struggling with addiction, becomes emotionally inconsistent—present one moment, withdrawn or volatile the next.

For children ages three to eight, whose cognitive development hasn't yet equipped them to understand that relationships can persist across distance or that adults have complex inner lives separate from parenting, these changes register as existential danger.

Research from the National Child Traumatic Stress Network shows us that children of parents with substance abuse issues face particularly acute attachment disruptions.

The unpredictability inherent in addiction—loving and engaged one day, absent or frightening the next—creates what clinicians call disorganized attachment, where children cannot develop coherent strategies for seeking comfort because they cannot predict whether their parent will provide safety or become a source of fear.

This unpredictability amplifies separation anxiety far beyond typical developmental levels, as children cannot trust that separation will end in reunion with a safe, regulated caregiver.

Regression represents one of the most visible manifestations of fear and attachment threat in young children. When a seven-year-old who has been dry at night for years suddenly begins wetting the bed, or when a five-year-old who spoke in full sentences reverts to baby talk, parents often feel alarmed or frustrated.

These behaviors, however, serve a psychological function: they represent an unconscious attempt to return to an earlier developmental stage when the child felt safer and more cared for. Regression says, "When I was smaller, my world was secure. Perhaps if I become small again, that security will return."

Here's something child development experts want you to know: regression during family transitions is nearly universal and typically temporary, resolving as children adjust to new routines and regain a sense of predictability. For neurodivergent children, however, regression may be more pronounced and persistent.

Children with autism spectrum disorder often show increased rigidity, more frequent meltdowns, or intensified repetitive behaviors when attachment security feels threatened. Children with ADHD may exhibit heightened impulsivity, emotional dysregulation, or difficulty with transitions that were previously manageable.

These responses reflect not weakness but the reality that neurodivergent children often have fewer regulatory resources available when stress increases.

The physical symptoms of fear—stomachaches before transitions between homes, headaches on mornings when a parent is expected but may not show up, difficulty sleeping when routines change—represent the body's response to chronic activation of the stress system.

Prolonged separation from primary attachment figures, particularly when combined with the chaos of parental addiction or high-conflict divorce, can impair children's developing capacity for emotional regulation. This means that the skills children need to manage difficult emotions become harder to build precisely when those emotions intensify.

Parents cannot eliminate their children's fear, but they can provide what attachment researchers call a "secure base"—consistent, predictable presence that communicates safety even amid change.

This requires not perfection but reliability in the small moments: showing up when promised, maintaining routines where possible, responding to distress with patience rather than dismissal, and offering reassurance through both words and physical presence that the child remains loved and protected regardless of what changes between adults.

If this sounds familiar, that's because it's meant to be. When stress is high, children—and adults—benefit from returning to the same grounding truths.

When Anger Shows Up: Recognizing Powerlessness, Loss of Control, and Healthy vs. Concerning Expressions of Rage

Anger in young children during divorce often catches parents off guard with its sudden intensity and seemingly disproportionate triggers.

A child who was previously easygoing may now explode over minor frustrations—the wrong plate at dinner, a sibling touching their toy, being asked to put on shoes.

These eruptions can feel personal, frightening, or exhausting, particularly when parents are already stretched thin managing their own emotions and the logistics of separation.

Yet anger in children ages three to eight during family transitions serves a critical psychological function: it represents an attempt to protest powerlessness and reclaim some sense of control in a world that has become unpredictable.

Developmental psychologists help us understand that young children have limited capacity to influence their environment through negotiation or problem-solving, leaving emotional expression as their primary tool for communicating distress.

When divorce disrupts the fundamental structures of their lives—who lives where, when they see each parent, whether routines remain consistent — children face a profound loss of control that adults may underestimate.

They cannot make parents reconcile, cannot choose their living arrangements, and cannot predict when changes will stop happening.

Anger becomes the language through which they say, "This isn't fair, I didn't choose this, and I need someone to hear how hard this is."

For children whose other parent struggles with addiction, anger may carry additional layers of confusion and betrayal.

A parent who is inconsistent, who breaks promises, or who behaves unpredictably due to substance use creates a particularly destabilizing environment where children cannot develop reliable expectations.

The anger that emerges reflects not only the divorce itself but the ongoing experience of disappointment and the child's inability to make that parent show up reliably or act safely.

Distinguishing between healthy expressions of anger and concerning escalations requires attention to both intensity and duration. Healthy anger in young children typically appears as brief outbursts—tantrums that peak and then resolve within twenty to thirty minutes, verbal protests that respond to comfort and validation, or physical expressions like stomping or throwing soft objects that don't cause harm.

These episodes allow children to release emotional pressure and often lead to moments of connection when parents respond with calm presence rather than punishment. A four-year-old who screams "I hate this!" about moving between houses, then accepts a hug and calms down, is processing grief in a developmentally normal way.

Concerning expressions of rage, by contrast, show patterns that suggest a child is overwhelmed beyond their capacity to regulate.

These include prolonged episodes that escalate rather than resolve, aggression directed at people or pets, self-harm behaviors like head-banging or hitting themselves, or rage that appears disconnected from identifiable triggers and erupts throughout daily life.

When anger becomes the dominant emotional state rather than one feeling among many, or when a child seems frightened by their own intensity, professional support becomes necessary.

Children with neurodevelopmental differences may express anger differently or with greater intensity due to differences in sensory processing, emotional regulation, and communication.

A child with autism may have meltdowns that look like rage but actually represent sensory or emotional overwhelm, requiring different responses than typical tantrums.

Children with ADHD often experience emotional dysregulation that makes anger feel more explosive and harder to control, even when the underlying cause is relatively minor.

Parents of children with neurodevelopmental differences benefit from learning their child's specific patterns—what precedes anger, what helps them regulate, and how to distinguish meltdowns from intentional defiance.

Responding to children's anger with validation rather than dismissal helps them feel heard without reinforcing destructive behavior.

Simple language like "You're really mad that you have to leave Mommy's house" or "It's okay to feel angry about this" acknowledges the emotion while maintaining boundaries around safety.

Creating opportunities for physical release—running, jumping, tearing paper, squeezing playdough—gives children acceptable outlets for the energy anger generates in their bodies.

Making Sense of Confusion: How Limited Cognitive Development Shapes Children's Understanding and Misunderstanding of Divorce

Confusion in young children during divorce stems not from insufficient explanation but from fundamental limitations in how their developing brains process abstract concepts, time, and causation.

Children ages three to eight are concrete thinkers who interpret the world through immediate, observable experiences rather than logical reasoning.

When parents separate, children face a concept—divorce—that exists beyond their cognitive capacity to fully comprehend, leaving them to construct their own explanations that are often frightening and inaccurate.

Developmental psychologists call this period one of **egocentrism**—a stage where children believe the world revolves around them and that their thoughts, wishes, or behaviors directly cause events.

This cognitive stage creates a particularly painful misunderstanding: children frequently believe they caused the divorce. If they argued with a parent, wished their parents would stop fighting, or misbehaved before the separation, they may conclude that their actions triggered the family's dissolution.

Research consistently demonstrates that children tend to internalize feelings of guilt and self-blame that can persist well into adulthood when not addressed through clear, repeated reassurance.

Preschoolers, ages two to five, face the most profound confusion. They are too young to grasp the meaning of divorce itself and often become fearful of losing their other parent as well. Their limited understanding of permanence means they may believe parents will remarry each other, reflecting magical thinking that wishes can reverse reality.

This age group also struggles with time perception in ways that intensify their distress. They cannot comprehend extended separations or understand schedules involving prolonged absences from a parent. Each goodbye feels potentially permanent because they lack the cognitive tools to reassure themselves that reunion will occur.

A landmark study published in *BMJ Pediatrics Open* looked at developmental outcomes in over, children ages three to five and found that those from divorced families showed statistically lower scores in overall development compared to children from intact families. The domains most strongly affected were social and emotional skills, physical health, and reading ability.

This research underscores that confusion during divorce isn't merely emotional—it has measurable impacts across multiple developmental areas, including cognitive abilities.

Children's confusion manifests behaviorally when they cannot articulate what they don't understand.

Signs of cognitive overwhelm include increased clinginess, fear of separations, tantrums, sleep disturbances, and eating problems. Some children become withdrawn and isolated, while others exhibit aggression or defiance.

Preschoolers may regress developmentally, losing previously mastered skills like toilet training or independent sleep. These behavioral changes represent attempts to communicate emotions and questions children lack the vocabulary and cognitive framework to express verbally.

For children with neurodevelopmental differences, cognitive confusion during divorce often intensifies.

Children with autism spectrum disorder may struggle even more with abstract concepts and show distress through increased rigidity, more frequent meltdowns, or withdrawal into repetitive behaviors that provide predictability.

Children with ADHD, already challenged by executive functioning difficulties, may find it nearly impossible to organize their understanding of family changes, leading to heightened impulsivity and emotional dysregulation.

Parents cannot accelerate their child's cognitive development, but they can provide explanations that match where the child actually is developmentally rather than where adults wish they could be.

This means avoiding abstract language like "irreconcilable differences" or "growing apart" in favor of concrete, simple statements: "Mommy and Daddy are going to live in different houses, but we both still love you very much."

It means repeating these explanations frequently, because young children need multiple exposures to integrate new information. And it means explicitly stating what children cannot infer on their own: "This is not your fault. Nothing you did or said made this happen. You are safe, and both of us will take care of you."

The confusion young kids face during divorce reflects genuine cognitive limitations, not emotional immaturity or resistance. Understanding this distinction helps parents respond with patience rather than frustration when children ask the same questions repeatedly or seem unable to grasp explanations that feel clear to adults.

Building the Foundation of Safety: Practical Strategies for Helping Children Feel Emotionally Secure Through Presence, Routine, and Responsive Attention

Safety for young children isn't built through grand gestures or perfect circumstances—it emerges from the small, repeated moments that anchor their days and communicate that someone is paying attention, that the world has structure, and that their feelings matter.

When divorce disrupts the foundation of family life, parents can rebuild a sense of security through three interconnected practices: consistent presence, predictable routines, and responsive attentions to children's emotional cues. These strategies work together to create what attachment researchers call a "secure base"—the felt sense that a child is protected and valued even when circumstances change.

Presence means more than physical proximity; it requires quality attention that signals to children they remain a priority despite adult upheaval.

Research on attachment security shows us that children regulate their emotions through connection with calm, available caregivers who notice their distress and respond with warmth.

For children ages three to eight, presence looks like sitting at eye level during conversations, putting away phones during transitions between homes, and creating brief but focused rituals of connection—ten minutes of undivided attention at bedtime, a special goodbye routine before school, or a consistent check-in after visits with the other parent.

These moments don't require elaborate planning or extended time; they require intentionality and the message that "I see you, I'm here, and you matter."

When a parent struggles with addiction, the other parent's consistent presence becomes even more critical. Children who experience unpredictability from one caregiver need the other to be reliably available, both physically and emotionally.

This doesn't mean perfection—parents will have hard days, moments of distraction, or times when their own stress makes full presence difficult.

What matters is the pattern over time: showing up when promised, following through on commitments, and repairing moments of disconnection rather than pretending they didn't happen.

Routine provides the external structure that young children's developing nervous systems cannot yet generate internally. Predictable schedules around meals, sleep, transitions, and play create islands of stability in what may otherwise feel like chaos.

Child development experts remind us that routines reduce anxiety by helping children anticipate what comes next, which allows them to relax rather than remaining in a constant state of vigilance.

A consistent morning sequence—breakfast, getting dressed, brushing teeth in the same order—builds competence and calm.

A predictable bedtime routine signals safety and helps regulate the sleep disruptions common during divorce.

Ideally, parents maintain similar routines across both households, creating continuity that helps children move between homes with less distress.

When co-parenting cooperation isn't possible, the parent providing primary stability can still establish reliable patterns within their own home.

Even when routines must shift due to changing circumstances, maintaining certain anchors—the same bedtime story, a particular song during car rides, a weekly pizza night—gives children touchstones they can count on.

For children with neurodevelopmental differences, routines serve an even more essential function. Children with autism often rely on predictability to manage sensory input and emotional regulation; unexpected changes can trigger meltdowns that reflect genuine overwhelm rather than defiance.

Children with ADHD benefit from external structure that compensates for executive functioning challenges. Visual schedules, transition warnings, and consistent sequences help these children navigate divorce-related changes with less dysregulation.

Responsive attention means noticing children's emotional signals and reflecting them back with empathy and validation.

When a four-year-old melts down over a minor frustration, an attuned parent recognizes the tantrum as communication about bigger fears and responds with "You're having such big feelings right now—I'm here with you" rather than punishment or dismissal.

When a seven-year-old grows quiet and withdrawn after a cancelled visit, attunement looks like sitting nearby and offering gentle observations: "You seem sad. It's okay to feel disappointed when plans change."

Attunement doesn't require parents to fix every problem or eliminate all distress. It requires witnessing children's experiences without minimizing them, naming emotions to help children develop emotional literacy, and staying present through difficult feelings rather than rushing to make them disappear.

This practice teaches children that their emotions are manageable and that they don't have to face overwhelming feelings alone—lessons that build resilience far beyond the immediate crisis of divorce.

The big feelings your child carries during divorce—fear, anger, confusion, and the urgent need for safety—are not signs of permanent damage or evidence that you've failed them. They are normal, developmentally appropriate responses to significant change, and they represent your child's attempt to communicate what they cannot yet fully understand or articulate.

When your five-year-old clings to your leg at drop-off or your seven-year-old explodes over a broken crayon, they are telling you something important: their world feels uncertain, and they need help finding their footing again.

Understanding the developmental roots of these emotions changes how parents can respond. Fear in young children reflects genuine threats to attachment security—the biological imperative to remain close to caregivers who ensure survival.

Anger emerges as protest against powerlessness, a child's way of saying "I didn't choose this, and I need someone to hear how hard it is."

Confusion stems from cognitive limitations that make abstract concepts like divorce impossible for young minds to grasp fully, leaving children to construct their own frightening explanations.

Beneath all of these responses lies the fundamental need to feel safe—not just physically protected, but emotionally held and relationally secure.

For children with neurodevelopmental differences and those who are highly sensitive, these emotional experiences often arrive with amplified intensity and require adapted responses. A child with autism may show distress through increased rigidity or withdrawal into repetitive behaviors.

A child with ADHD may become more impulsive and emotionally explosive as their already-challenged regulation systems become further taxed.

Recognizing these patterns as communication rather than defiance allows parents to respond with strategies that match their child's actual needs.

The practical tools for building safety—consistent presence, predictable routines, and attuned responses—work together to create the foundation of safety children need during family transitions.

These strategies don't require perfection or ideal circumstances. They require intentionality in small moments: sitting at eye level during difficult conversations, maintaining bedtime rituals even when schedules shift, noticing when a child grows quiet after a cancelled visit and offering gentle validation rather than forced cheerfulness.

Safety emerges from patterns over time, from the accumulation of moments when a child's distress is met with presence rather than dismissal.

When one parent struggles with addiction, the other parent's role in providing this consistent foundation becomes even more critical. Children who experience unpredictability from one caregiver need the other to be reliably available, both physically and emotionally.

This doesn't mean eliminating all difficult feelings or shielding children from every disappointment—it means staying present through the hard moments and helping children understand that their emotions are manageable and that they don't have to face overwhelming feelings alone.

Parents cannot prevent their children from experiencing fear, anger, or confusion during divorce. These emotions are part of the landscape of significant change, and attempting to eliminate them entirely would require denying reality.

What parents can do—and what matters profoundly—is help children move through these feelings with support rather than in isolation.

When children learn that their big emotions can be witnessed, named, and survived with a caring adult nearby, they develop resilience that extends far beyond the immediate crisis of family transition.

Your child's big feelings are invitations for connection, not evidence of your failure. You have the capacity to answer those invitations with the steadiness they need, even on days when you don't feel steady yourself.

The foundation of safety you're building through presence, routine, and attuned response will serve your child not only through divorce but throughout their development—teaching them that they are worthy of care, that their emotions matter, and that they can trust the adults in their lives to show up even when things are hard.

CHAPTER 4

Finding the Right Words

How to Talk With Children Honestly and Kindly

You've rehearsed the conversation a dozen times in your head, searching for words that will somehow make this easier for your child to hear. Each version feels wrong—too much information, not enough truth, too scary, too vague — and the weight of getting it right sits heavy in your chest. The truth is, there are no perfect words for telling a child that their family is changing. But there are words that help, words that offer clarity without overwhelming, honesty without fear, and truth wrapped in reassurance that they are loved and safe.

Many parents worry that talking directly about divorce will make it more real or more painful for their children. The opposite is often true. Children are already sensing the tension, noticing the changes, and filling in the blanks with their powerful imaginations—and what they imagine is frequently worse than reality.

A four-year-old who overhears hushed arguments may believe she caused them.

When parents suddenly announce that Daddy is moving out without explanation, a six-year-old may assume something terrible happened that no one trusts him enough to share. A seven-year-old watching her mother cry might conclude that the whole world is falling apart.

Silence doesn't protect children from pain. It leaves them alone with their confusion and fear, without the tools to make sense of what's happening around them.

This chapter offers you language—not scripts to memorize and recite perfectly, but frameworks and examples that can guide your conversations with your child in ways that match their developmental stage and emotional needs.

You'll find concrete phrases for that first difficult conversation when you tell your child about the separation, along with guidance for what to include and what to leave out. You'll discover how to answer the questions that follow, some asked directly and some hidden in behavior or play: *Why are you getting divorced? Is it my fault? Do you still love each other? Do you still love me? Where will I live? Will I still see both of you?*

The goal isn't to eliminate your child's sadness or confusion—those feelings are natural and valid responses to real loss and change. The goal is to help your child feel informed enough to understand their changing world while protected from information that creates unnecessary fear or asks them to carry adult emotional burdens.

This means finding the balance between honesty and developmentally appropriate boundaries, between acknowledging hard truths and offering steady reassurance.

You'll also find guidance for what not to say—the phrases and explanations that, despite good intentions, can burden children with blame, force them to choose sides, or expose them to adult conflicts and details they're not equipped to process.

Even in your pain, even when your ex-partner's behavior feels impossible to explain neutrally, your child needs to hear about the divorce in ways that don't ask them to be your confidant, your ally against the other parent, or the keeper of adult secrets.

Special attention is given throughout this chapter to adapting your communication for children at different points in the 3-8 age range, recognizing that a three-year-old needs far simpler, more specific language than an eight-year-old who can grasp more complexity.

You'll also find strategies for supporting children with neurodevelopmental differences who may need more literal explanations, visual aids, or repeated conversations to process what they're hearing, as well as guidance for navigating conversations when one parent's addiction or concerning behavior makes simple explanations feel impossible.

You don't need to have all the answers right now or explain everything perfectly in one conversation. What matters most is that you begin—that you offer your child the gift of truth delivered with love, the reassurance that their questions are welcome, and the steady message that no matter what changes, your love for them never will.

The First Conversation: What to Say When You Tell Your Child About the Divorce—Simple Scripts for Different Ages and Situations

The first conversation about divorce works best when both parents can deliver the news together in a calm, neutral moment—ideally not during a transition time like before school or bedtime, and not in the immediate aftermath of a heated argument when emotions are still raw.

Child development experts emphasize that children benefit from seeing both parents present a united front on this single message: the marriage is ending, but the parenting partnership continues, and your child's security remains intact. When both parents participate, it reduces your child's fear that one parent is disappearing entirely and minimizes the risk that the child will hear conflicting or blame-filled versions of events from each parent separately.

However, many parents reading this are navigating divorces where cooperative communication feels impossible. If the other parent refuses to participate, is actively using substances, or would use the conversation as an opportunity to blame or create conflict in front of the child, it may be healthier for one parent to have this conversation alone. In these situations, the speaking parent can still use inclusive language—"Your mom and I have decided" rather than "I decided"—while keeping the focus on facts and reassurance rather than blame.

For children ages three to five, the initial conversation should last no more than five minutes and use the simplest possible language tied to concrete realities the child can observe. Preschoolers think in very literal terms and struggle with abstract concepts like "growing apart" or "not in love anymore." They need to hear what will change in their daily life and what will stay the same.

A parent might say: "Mommy and Daddy are not going to live in the same house anymore. You will have a home with Mommy and a home with Daddy. We both love you very much. This is not your fault. Nothing you did made this happen."

Repetition matters enormously at this age, as the child will likely not absorb or retain much from the first conversation. Parents should expect to revisit these same simple messages many times in the days and weeks that follow.

Pairing the conversation with a children's book specifically about divorce—such as *Two Homes* by Claire Masurel, which shows a child with two loving homes that share similarities—can provide a visual anchor and normalize the experience.

For children ages six to eight, parents can offer slightly more information while still maintaining clear boundaries around adult details. School-age children have greater cognitive capacity to understand that relationships can change and that parents can make decisions that affect the whole family. They're also more likely to ask direct questions and to worry about logistics.

A parent might say: "Dad and I have decided to get a divorce. That means we won't be married anymore and we'll live in different houses. We've been unhappy together for a while, and we think this is the best decision for our family. It is absolutely not your fault—nothing you did or didn't do caused this. We will always be your parents, and we both love you just as much as we always have. You'll spend time with both of us, and we'll make a schedule so you always know what's happening."

At this age, children often harbor unspoken fears about being abandoned, having to choose between parents, or losing their home, school, and friends. Proactively addressing these concerns—even before the child asks—can prevent weeks of silent worry. Parents can add: "You'll still go to the same school. You'll still see your friends. You'll still have all your toys and your room. We're going to make sure you feel safe and loved no matter what."

Throughout these conversations, parents should watch for the child's emotional capacity and be prepared to pause if the child becomes overwhelmed, offering comfort and the promise to talk more later when they're ready.

Answering the Questions That Follow: Responding to 'Why?' 'Is It My Fault?' and Other Worries Children Express Directly and Indirectly

After the initial conversation about divorce, children rarely process everything in one sitting. Instead, questions emerge gradually—some asked directly over breakfast or at bedtime, others revealed through worried behavior, repetitive play themes, or sudden emotional outbursts that seem disconnected from the moment.

Parents who expect a single conversation to resolve their child's confusion often find themselves caught off guard weeks later when new worries surface, or when the same questions return again and again despite having been answered before.

When both parents participate, it reduces your child's fear that one parent is disappearing entirely and minimizes the risk that the child will hear conflicting or blame-filled versions of events from each parent separately.

The question "Why are you getting divorced?" appears simple on the surface, but it carries different meanings depending on the child's age and what they're truly asking underneath. A four-year-old asking "why" may be seeking a concrete reason tied to something observable—*Did someone do something bad? Did something break?*—while a seven-year-old may be searching for logic that helps them predict whether other relationships in their life might also end.

Developmental psychologists emphasize that the most helpful responses focus on the parental relationship rather than individual blame, using language like "Mommy and Daddy weren't happy together anymore and we decided it's better for our family if we live in separate homes" rather than detailed explanations about specific conflicts or failures.

For very young children, repeating the same simple answer multiple times without frustration communicates safety more effectively than elaborate explanations.

Preschoolers often need to hear the same information dozens of times before it begins to feel real and manageable. Their developing brains process big changes slowly, and repetition is how they build understanding and reduce anxiety.

The worry "Is it my fault?" represents one of the most painful and persistent fears children carry during divorce.

Research in child psychology consistently shows that young children are egocentric in their thinking—they naturally assume they are the center of most events happening around them.

A five-year-old who remembers her parents arguing after she spilled juice may genuinely believe her accident caused the divorce. A six-year-old who was told to be quiet during a tense moment may conclude that his noise destroyed the marriage. Even when parents have explicitly said "This is not your fault," children often need to hear this message repeated in multiple contexts before they truly internalize it.

Parents can respond to this worry by saying clearly and directly: "Divorce is never a child's fault. This is about grown-up problems between Mommy and Daddy. Nothing you did, nothing you said, and nothing you didn't do caused this to happen. We love you exactly the same as we always have."

When children ask this question repeatedly, it's not because they didn't hear the answer—it's because the fear is so big that it needs multiple reassurances before it begins to shrink.

Some worries children carry never get asked aloud. A child who suddenly refuses to go to preschool may be afraid that if she leaves her parent, that parent will disappear like the other one did. A child who begins hoarding food in his room may be worried that resources are no longer secure.

A child who repeatedly asks "Do you still love me?" in different ways—through clinginess, attention-seeking behavior, or testing boundaries—is seeking evidence that love remains constant even when family structure has changed.

Parents can address these indirect worries by naming what they observe and offering reassurance without waiting for the question.

"I notice you've been worried about me leaving. I will always come back. I will always be your mom."

Or, "You seem scared about going to Dad's house this weekend. It's okay to feel nervous about changes. Dad loves you and you'll be safe there, and I'll be right here when you come home."

Children with neurodevelopmental differences may express worries in less typical ways or need more concrete, repeated explanations.

A child with autism might ask the same question dozens of times not because they don't understand the answer, but because the ritual of asking and hearing the response provides regulation and comfort.

A child with ADHD might show worry through increased hyperactivity or impulsivity rather than words.

Meeting children where they are—answering the same question patiently each time, providing visual schedules that show when they'll see each parent, offering sensory comfort during difficult conversations—honors their unique processing needs while delivering the same core message: *You are loved. This is not your fault. You are safe.*

What Not to Say: Avoiding Blame, Adult Details, False Promises, and Language That Burdens Children with Adult Pain

In the rawness of divorce, when emotions run high and hurt feels overwhelming, certain phrases can slip out that seem harmless in the moment but carry weight that children are not equipped to bear.

The words parents choose—or avoid—during this transition shape not only how children understand the divorce, but how they understand themselves, their worth, and their place in both parents' lives.

Developmental psychologists consistently emphasize that protecting children from blame, adult details, false promises, and language saturated with parental pain is not about dishonesty; it's about developmentally appropriate boundaries that preserve childhood while honoring truth.

Avoiding blame means resisting the urge to cast one parent as the villain, even when that parent's behavior feels unforgivable.

Phrases like "Your father chose his drinking over us" or "Mommy cares more about her new boyfriend than our family" force children into an impossible position.

Research in child development shows that children ages 3-8 are deeply attached to both parents and experience criticism of one parent as an attack on part of themselves.

When a parent says "Your dad ruined everything," a young child hears "Half of who you are is bad."

Even when one parent's actions directly caused the divorce—through infidelity, addiction, or abandonment—children benefit from neutral explanations that acknowledge the marriage ended without requiring them to judge or reject a parent they still love.

This doesn't mean lying or pretending harmful behavior doesn't exist. It means separating the parent's actions from the child's relationship with that parent, and offering developmentally appropriate truth without editorial commentary.

Instead of "Your mom left because she's selfish," a parent might say, "Your mom and I couldn't agree on important things, and we decided it's better for everyone if we live separately." The child's experience of the other parent's behavior will speak for itself over time; they don't need a parent's anger added to their own confusion.

Sharing adult details —the specifics of affairs, financial betrayals, or intimate relationship failures—overwhelms children's cognitive and emotional capacity.

A six-year-old who hears "Daddy had a girlfriend while he was still married to me" now carries information they cannot process, cannot fix, and should never have been asked to hold.

Family therapists note that exposing children to these details often serves the speaking parent's need to be understood or vindicated rather than the child's need for clarity. Young children don't need to know why the marriage failed in adult terms; they need to know that both parents still love them and that the divorce was not their fault.

False promises emerge from a parent's desire to ease immediate pain, but they create deeper wounds when reality fails to match the reassurance.

Telling a child "Everything will be exactly the same" when their entire world is changing, or "Maybe Mommy and Daddy will get back together someday" when reconciliation isn't possible, sets children up for prolonged hope followed by crushing disappointment.

Child psychologists emphasize that children are remarkably resilient when given honest information paired with reassurance about what will remain stable. A more helpful approach acknowledges change while emphasizing continuity: "Some things will be different, like having two homes. But some very important things will stay the same—we both love you, you'll still go to your school, and you'll still see both of us."

Language that burdens children with adult pain—statements like "I don't know how I'll survive this" or "You're the only reason I'm still here" — places children in the role of emotional caretaker, a position that disrupts healthy development and creates anxiety.

When parents share their devastation, rage, or despair with young children, those children often conclude they must fix their parent's pain or hide their own feelings to avoid adding to the burden. Children need to see that their parents have adult support systems and can manage difficult emotions without requiring the child's comfort or solutions.

Adapting Your Words: Communication Strategies for Neurodivergent Children and Those Who Need Concrete, Visual, or Repeated Explanations

Neurodivergent children—including those with autism spectrum disorder, ADHD, sensory processing differences, or other cognitive variations—often experience divorce-related conversations with heightened intensity and unique processing needs that require parents to adapt their communication approach significantly.

Research in developmental psychology shows that children who think more concretely, process language literally, or rely heavily on routine and predictability may struggle with the abstract emotional concepts and ambiguous explanations that neurotypical children can navigate more easily.

When a parent says "We're growing apart," a child with autism may picture their parents physically expanding and moving away from each other. When a parent explains "Sometimes people fall out of love," a child who thinks literally may become terrified that love is something you can accidentally drop and lose.

Developmental psychologists emphasize that children with neurodevelopmental differences benefit most from **clear, direct, and concrete language** that describes observable facts rather than emotional abstractions.

Instead of "Mommy and Daddy aren't happy together anymore," a more effective approach might be: "Mommy and Daddy have decided to live in two different houses. You will spend some nights at Mommy's house and some nights at Daddy's house. We will make a schedule, so you always know where you'll be sleeping."

This language removes ambiguity, provides concrete information about what will change, and offers predictability—all critical elements for children whose nervous systems rely on structure to feel safe.

Visual supports serve as essential tools for children who process information better through images than through verbal explanation alone.

Marriage and family therapists working with neurodivergent children recommend creating visual schedules that show the child's week using pictures, colors, or symbols to represent which parent they'll be with each day.

A calendar with photos of each parent's house, marked clearly with "Monday: Mom's house" and "Tuesday: Mom's house" and "Wednesday: Dad's house," provides a concrete reference point the child can return to repeatedly without needing to ask or remember verbal information.

Social stories—short, personalized narratives with simple text and photos that walk through exactly what will happen during transitions—help prepare children for changes in routine by rehearsing the sequence of events before they occur.

Repetition without frustration becomes particularly important for children who need to hear the same information multiple times before it feels real and manageable.

A child with ADHD may ask "When am I going to Dad's house?" dozens of times not because they didn't hear or understand the answer, but because their working memory makes it difficult to hold onto information, or because the anxiety of the change requires repeated reassurance.

Child psychologists note that parents can support this need by answering the question calmly each time, pointing to the visual schedule, and offering the same consistent response: "You're going to Dad's house on Friday after school. Let's look at the calendar together."

Neurodivergent children may also express their worries and confusion through behavior rather than words, particularly when language processing or emotional expression feels overwhelming.

A child who cannot articulate "I'm scared about the divorce" may instead show increased stimming behaviors, meltdowns over seemingly small changes, refusal to transition between activities, or regression in self-care skills.

Parents can support these children by naming what they observe without requiring verbal response: "I notice you're having a hard time right now. Big changes can feel scary. You are safe. I am here with you."

Sensory considerations matter significantly during difficult conversations. Conducting divorce-related discussions in a quiet, low-stimulation environment—away from bright lights, loud noises, or chaotic spaces—helps children regulate enough to process what they're hearing.

Offering sensory tools like fidget objects, weighted blankets, or noise-canceling headphones during conversations honors the reality that some children listen and process better when their bodies have something regulating to do.

Parents navigating divorce with neurodivergent children benefit from working closely with therapists, school counselors, or developmental specialists who understand their child's specific processing needs and can help create individualized communication plans that respect both the truth of the family's situation and the child's unique way of understanding their world.

Finding the right words to talk with your child about divorce is not about achieving perfection or delivering a flawless script that erases all confusion and pain. It's about offering your child the gift of truth delivered with love, the reassurance that their questions matter, and the steady message that even as family structure changes, your commitment to them never wavers.

The conversations outlined in this chapter—whether the first difficult explanation of separation, the repeated reassurances that the divorce isn't their fault, or the careful navigation of questions about a parent's addiction or absence—are not one-time events but ongoing dialogues that will evolve as your child grows and their understanding deepens.

Research in child development consistently shows that children who receive developmentally appropriate, honest information about divorce paired with consistent emotional support navigate family transitions with greater resilience than children left to fill in the blanks with their imaginations or piece together fragments from overheard arguments.

The words you choose create a framework through which your child interprets not only the divorce itself, but their own worth, their safety in the world, and their right to love both parents without shame or divided loyalty.

When parents communicate with clarity and compassion—naming the change while emphasizing continuity, acknowledging hard feelings while offering reassurance—they provide children with an anchor in turbulent waters.

The guidance in this chapter recognizes that many parents are navigating these conversations alone, without the cooperation of an ex-partner who might share the emotional labor of explanation or present a united front.

Even in these circumstances, the parent providing stability can still offer their child truthful, developmentally appropriate information that protects them from blame and adult burdens. You don't need your ex-partner's participation to speak to your child with honesty and care.

The principles that matter most across all divorce-related conversations include:

- Keeping explanations simple, concrete, and focused on observable changes rather than abstract emotional concepts that overwhelm young children's cognitive capacity
- Repeating core messages—this is not your fault, we both love you, you are safe—as many times as your child needs to hear them, recognizing that repetition builds understanding and reduces anxiety
- Protecting children from blame, adult details, and language that asks them to choose sides or carry emotional burdens they're not developmentally equipped to manage
- Adapting communication for children with neurodevelopmental differences through visual aids, literal language, and patience with processing differences that require more concrete or repeated explanations

For children with neurodevelopmental differences, the strategies in this chapter emphasize meeting children where they are—using visual schedules, personalized narratives, and sensory-aware approaches that honor their unique ways of understanding the world.

These adaptations aren't accommodations that water down truth; they're bridges that make truth accessible to children whose brains work beautifully but differently.

You will not get every conversation right. There will be moments when emotions override careful planning, when your child asks a question you don't know how to answer, or when the words that seemed clear in your head come out tangled and insufficient.

What matters is not perfection but presence—your willingness to show up, to listen, to repair when conversations go sideways, and to keep the door open for questions that will emerge gradually over months and years rather than all at once.

Words alone, however, cannot carry the full weight of helping your child through divorce. The next chapter turns from words to the daily practices that reinforce what you've communicated—the routines, rituals, and moments of repair that help children feel safe even when their world has changed.

CHAPTER 5

Creating Safety in Everyday Moments

Routines, Reassurance, and Emotional Repair

Up to this point, we've focused on understanding what children feel and why. In this chapter, we turn toward how safety is rebuilt in daily life—through routines, repair, and the small moments that quietly restore trust.

Safety, for a young child, isn't an abstract concept or a feeling they can name — it lives in the small, repeated moments that shape their days.

It's found in the familiar rhythm of breakfast before school, the predictable goodbye routine at drop-off, the certainty that bedtime will unfold the same gentle way it did the night before.

These ordinary moments become extraordinary anchors when a child's world has shifted in ways they don't fully understand. Ideas in this chapter may sound familiar because they are. It's beneficial for both children and adults to return to the same anchoring facts when they are experiencing high levels of stress.

When parents separate, the ground beneath a child's feet can feel suddenly unsteady. The home they knew may change, and the people they love most now live in different places. Schedules shift, belongings travel back and forth, and the predictable flow of daily life gets disrupted in ways both large and small.

For young children who are still developing their sense of time, cause and effect, and emotional regulation, these changes can feel overwhelming—not because anything catastrophic has happened, but because the reliable patterns that helped them feel secure have been altered.

This chapter focuses on something entirely within your control, even when so much else feels uncertain: the power of everyday moments to rebuild and maintain your child's sense of safety.

You don't need a perfect co-parenting relationship to create stability for your child. You don't need two identical households or a cooperative ex-partner to establish routines that help your child feel grounded.

What you need is an understanding of why predictability matters so deeply to young nervous systems, and practical strategies for building that predictability into the daily life you share with your child.

Research in child development and attachment consistently shows that children regulate their emotions and manage stress through shared regulation with their caregivers.

When the world feels unpredictable, children look to their parents' consistency and calm presence as proof that they're still safe.

Bruce Perry emphasizes that steady, predictable experiences can help children regain a sense of calm and emotional safety when life feels overwhelming. For neurodivergent children—especially those with autism or ADHD who often find comfort in routine—this predictability can provide an important foundation for feeling secure during transitions and sensory challenges.

But what happens when you lose your patience? When you snap at your child because you're exhausted and overwhelmed? When they witness tension between you and their other parent, or when you can't control what happens during visits to the other household?

This chapter also introduces the concept of emotional repair—the practice of reconnecting with your child after moments of rupture, stress, or disconnection. Repair is one of the most powerful tools available to parents navigating divorce, because it teaches children that relationships can withstand conflict and that mistakes don't mean the end of love or safety.

You will have hard days when you feel like you're failing, and you may not always respond the way you wish you had. None of this means you're damaging your child. What matters most isn't perfection—it's your willingness to show up consistently, to notice when your child needs reassurance, and to reconnect when things go sideways.

In the pages ahead, you'll find concrete strategies for establishing routines that work in your specific situation, recognizing when your child is seeking connection even when they can't ask for it directly, and practicing repair in ways that are developmentally appropriate for young children.

You'll learn how to build small rituals of safety into ordinary moments—rituals that communicate to your child, again and again, that they are loved, that you are present, and that even though things have changed, they can count on you to be their steady place in an uncertain world.

The Power of Predictability: Why Routines Matter for Children's Nervous Systems and Sense of Security During Divorce

When a child's world shifts through divorce, their nervous system responds before their mind can make sense of what's happening.

The automatic nervous system—the part of the body that operates beneath conscious awareness—constantly scans the environment for signals of safety or threat.

Polyvagal Theory, developed by Stephen Porges, highlights how children often rely on predictability as a signal of safety. When routines shift or become less consistent, children may feel unsettled or anxious, as their bodies are still learning how to adjust to change.

This biological response isn't something children choose or control—it's hardwired into their development. Their developing brains, particularly the prefrontal cortex responsible for emotional regulation and impulse control, remain immature throughout early childhood.

Without the cognitive tools to reason through uncertainty or reassure themselves that change doesn't equal danger, young children rely heavily on external cues—primarily the predictable presence and responses of their caregivers—to determine whether they're safe, which means that when routines vanish, children lose one of their primary sources of reassurance.

The stress of unpredictability activates what researchers call survival mode, a state in which a child's nervous system prioritizes immediate safety over connection, learning, or play. Parents may notice this shift through physical symptoms like headaches, stomachaches, or sleep disturbances.

Emotional changes often appear as well—increased tantrums, heightened sensitivity to small frustrations, difficulty concentrating, or withdrawal from activities the child once enjoyed. Behavioral changes such as regression to earlier developmental stages, defiance, or struggles with transitions between activities or locations all signal a nervous system working overtime to manage perceived threat.

For neurodivergent children, particularly those with autism or ADHD, the impact of disrupted routines intensifies significantly. These children often depend on predictable patterns to manage sensory input, navigate transitions, and maintain emotional regulation.

When divorce dismantles established routines, neurodivergent children may experience more severe dysregulation, longer recovery times from upsets, and heightened difficulty adapting to new schedules or environments.

Consistent routines function as a direct antidote to this nervous system stress. When a child experiences the same bedtime ritual night after night, the same morning sequence before school, the same predictable goodbye and reunion with their parent, their body receives repeated messages of safety.

These patterns don't need to be elaborate or perfect—what matters is their consistency. A simple routine of reading two books, singing the same song, and saying the same goodnight phrase becomes a powerful signal that despite the changes in their family, some things remain stable and trustworthy.

Research on children's stress responses shows that structured, predictable environments directly support emotional regulation and reduce anxiety. When routines remain consistent across both households—similar bedtimes, mealtimes, homework expectations, and screen time rules—children experience fewer jarring transitions between homes.

This consistency communicates that both parents remain committed to their wellbeing, even if the parents no longer live together.

The concept of co-regulation explains why parental consistency matters so profoundly. Children don't yet possess fully developed self-soothing capacities; instead, they borrow calm from their caregivers' regulated nervous systems.

When a parent maintains predictable routines even during stressful times, they offer their child both the external structure of the routine itself and the internal reassurance of the parent's steady presence.

As therapist Deb Dana notes, nervous systems exist in constant conversation with one another—a parent's regulated state directly influences their child's ability to return to calm.

Routines don't eliminate the pain or confusion of divorce, but they create islands of safety in uncertain waters.

They tell a child's body, in the language it understands best, that they remain held, that their world still contains reliable patterns, and that their parent will show up consistently even when everything else has changed.

Building and Maintaining Routines Across Two Households: Practical Strategies When Co-Parenting Is Cooperative—and When It's Not

When co-parenting works cooperatively, establishing consistent routines across two households becomes a shared project—one that directly benefits your child.

Parents who can communicate effectively about schedules, expectations, and daily rhythms create a bridge between homes that helps children move back and forth with less disruption.

Research from the American Academy of Child and Adolescent Psychiatry shows that children adjust more successfully to divorce when parents maintain similar routines, bedtimes, meal patterns, and behavioral expectations across both households.

When parents can work together cooperatively, they have the opportunity to develop a detailed parenting plan that outlines not just custody schedules but also the daily structure of the child's life. This might include agreements about consistent bedtimes (perhaps 7:30 p.m. for a four-year-old in both homes), similar morning routines before school, aligned expectations around homework time for school-age children, and shared rules about screen time or treats.

When a child knows that bedtime follows the same sequence of bath, books, and songs regardless of which parent's house they're in, their nervous system doesn't have to recalibrate each time they transition.

There are practical tools that can support this consistency.

Shared calendars, co-parenting apps, or simple communication notebooks that travel with your child help parents stay informed about schedule changes, upcoming school events, or shifts in the child's needs.

Regular, child-focused check-ins between parents—whether weekly phone calls or monthly coffee meetings—create space to adjust routines as children grow and their needs change.

The reality, however, is that many parents reading this don't have a cooperative co-parenting relationship.

Perhaps the other parent dismisses the importance of routines, keeps irregular schedules, or actively resists any attempt at coordination. Communication may have broken down entirely, or the other parent's addiction or mental health struggles make consistency impossible in their household.

In these situations, parents often feel helpless, watching their child struggle with the whiplash of moving between vastly different environments.

Here's what I've learned matters most: you cannot control what happens in the other household, but you can create unwavering consistency in your own home. This unilateral consistency matters profoundly.

When a child experiences predictable routines in at least one environment, they have a secure base to return to, a place where their nervous system can settle even if the other home feels chaotic or unpredictable.

In high-conflict or non-cooperative situations, parents benefit from treating the legal parenting plan as the foundation.

Following it precisely provides both legal protection and predictability for the child. This means honoring pickup times, respecting the schedule, and documenting any violations. Beyond the formal schedule, focus on what you directly control: the rhythms and rituals of your own household.

Establish and maintain consistent routines for mornings, after school, mealtimes, homework, and bedtime in your home regardless of what happens elsewhere.

A seven-year-old who knows that in Mom's house, homework always happens at the kitchen table right after snack time, followed by thirty minutes of play before dinner, gains security from that pattern even if Dad's house operates differently.

The routine itself becomes a form of reassurance.

Set firm boundaries around communication with the other parent. Limit interactions to written formats—email or co-parenting apps—focused solely on logistics and the child's needs.

Avoid engaging in arguments about parenting approaches; instead, document concerns when necessary and consult with legal or therapeutic professionals rather than trying to change the other parent's behavior directly.

For neurologically different children who struggle intensely with transitions between different household expectations, visual schedules can help.

A simple chart showing what happens in each home—not as judgment but as information—gives the child a cognitive map. Some parents create a "transition object" that travels with the child, like a special stuffed animal or blanket, providing sensory continuity across environments.

Most importantly, resist the urge to compete or compensate.

Maintaining steady, boring consistency serves your child better than becoming the "fun parent" with fewer rules or the "strict parent" trying to counterbalance perceived laxness elsewhere. Your child needs your home to be predictable, not perfect.

Recognizing When Your Child Needs Reassurance: Reading Cues for Connection and Responding to Invisible Worries

Children rarely announce their worries directly.

A four-year-old doesn't walk up and say, "I'm afraid you'll stop loving me now that Daddy's gone."

A seven-year-old won't articulate, "I think the divorce happened because I was too loud." Instead, these invisible worries emerge through behavioral shifts, physical complaints, changes in play, and questions that seem simple on the surface but carry deeper fears underneath.

Learning to read these cues requires parents to become observers of patterns rather than waiting for explicit requests for help.

As Tina Payne Bryson explains, young children frequently communicate emotional distress through behavior because their emotional vocabulary is still developing. Feelings like confusion, fear, or guilt can be especially hard to express directly. When caregivers notice these indirect signals and respond with understanding, they create opportunities to reassure children before worries become overwhelming.

Behavioral cues often appear as changes in a child's baseline functioning.

A previously independent five-year-old who suddenly refuses to play alone in their room may be signaling fear of separation or abandonment.

Regression behaviors—bedwetting after months of dryness, thumb-sucking that had stopped, baby talk in a child who speaks clearly—frequently indicate that a child's sense of security has been shaken and they're seeking the comfort of earlier developmental stages when life felt safer.

Increased clinginess at drop-offs, resistance to going to the other parent's house, or excessive worry about a parent's whereabouts all communicate an underlying question: "Will you still be here when I need you?"

Physical complaints without medical explanation serve as another common channel for invisible worries. Stomachaches before transitions between homes, headaches on Sunday nights, or sudden fatigue when discussing family changes often mask emotional distress that the child cannot articulate.

Research from the American Academy of Pediatrics shows that children experiencing family stress frequently somaticize anxiety, expressing psychological discomfort through physical symptoms their bodies can name even when their minds cannot.

Changes in play patterns offer particularly valuable windows into children's internal worlds. A child who repeatedly crashes toy cars together, stages scenarios where dolls get left behind, or creates stories where families break apart and reunite is processing their experience through the symbolic language of play.

Garry Landreth highlights that play provides children with a natural and safe way to express feelings that may feel too confusing or frightening to verbalize. Repeated themes in play can reflect a child's ongoing effort to understand an experience, offering parents opportunities to respond with gentle reassurance and emotional support.

Beyond behavioral and physical cues, **questions disguised as observations** require careful listening.

When a six-year-old says, "Mommy seems sad a lot now," they're often asking, "Is Mommy okay? Did I make her sad? Will she be able to take care of me?"

When a child comments, "Daddy has a new apartment," they may be wondering, "Does he still want to be my daddy? Is there room for me there?"

These statements invite parents to look beneath the surface and respond to the unspoken concern.

Responding effectively doesn't require perfect words or therapeutic training.

It requires presence and validation.

When you notice a cue—your daughter clinging tighter at bedtime, your son asking for the third time if you'll pick him up from school—pause and acknowledge what you're observing: "I notice you want extra hugs tonight. Sometimes when things change, we need more closeness. I'm right here, and I'm not going anywhere."

For neurologically different children who may struggle to identify or communicate emotions, parents might need to name possibilities: "Some kids worry that divorce means a parent stops loving them. That's not true for you—both Mom and Dad love you just as much as always."

This direct approach provides language for feelings the child senses but cannot express.

The most powerful reassurance comes not from eliminating all worry but from teaching children that their concerns matter, that asking for comfort is safe, and that their parent will notice when they're struggling even when they can't find words to ask for help.

The Practice of Emotional Repair: How to Reconnect With Your Child After Hard Moments, Conflict Exposure, or Parental Stress

No parent navigates divorce without moments they wish they could take back.

The morning you snapped at your child because you were exhausted from another sleepless night worrying about finances.

The afternoon your five-year-old overheard a tense phone call with your ex and saw your face crumple with frustration.

The evening your child returned from a visit, and you couldn't hide your anger at broken promises or concerning behavior from the other household.

These ruptures in connection happen, and they don't mean you've failed your child. What matters profoundly is what happens next—the practice of emotional repair.

As Daniel Siegel explains, rupture and repair are normal experiences within close relationships. Children benefit not from flawless parenting, but from caregivers who can recognize moments of disconnection and make space for reconnection. These repair moments help children learn that love endures through mistakes, that big emotions can be navigated safely, and that their parent remains emotionally present even when things feel hard.

The process of repair begins with the parent's own regulation.

When you've lost patience, witnessed your child's distress after conflict exposure, or recognized that your stress has affected your responsiveness, the first step involves calming your own nervous system before approaching your child.

This might mean taking several deep breaths, stepping into another room briefly, or using a simple grounding technique like placing your hand on your heart and reminding yourself that repair is possible. You cannot offer your child co-regulation if you remain dysregulated yourself.

Once you've found even a small measure of calm, approach your child with gentle acknowledgment of what happened.

For young children ages three to five, simple language works best: "I got frustrated earlier and my voice got loud. That wasn't okay. Your body might have felt scared when I yelled."

For children ages six to eight, slightly more explanation helps: "I was feeling really stressed about grown-up things, and I didn't handle my feelings well. That wasn't fair to you, and I'm sorry."

Repair can take many forms, but it often includes simple gestures like acknowledging what happened, recognizing how the child may have felt, and reassuring them that your love and connection remain steady. As Tina Payne Bryson explains, these moments help children learn that mistakes are natural and that relationships grow stronger through honesty and reconnection.

Physical reconnection often completes the repair process for young children whose primary language is touch and presence rather than words.

After acknowledging what happened, offer a hug, invite your child to sit close, or engage in a brief shared activity that rebuilds connection—reading a favorite book together, playing a simple game, or taking a short walk.

For neurodivergent children who may need more time to process or who experience touch differently, respect their pace and offer connection in ways that feel safe to them, whether that's sitting nearby without touching or engaging in parallel play.

When children have been exposed to conflict between parents—an argument they overheard, tension they witnessed during an exchange, or distress they experienced after a difficult visit—repair requires additional reassurance.

Children often internalize parental conflict as evidence that they caused the problem or that their world is fundamentally unsafe. Clear, repeated messages help counter these fears: "The argument you heard was between the grown-ups. It wasn't about you, and it wasn't your fault. You are safe, and both Mom and Dad love you."

Repair doesn't erase the hard moment, but it prevents that moment from becoming a lasting wound. It transforms rupture into an opportunity for your child to learn that relationships can weather storms, that feelings can be acknowledged and worked through, and that your love remains constant even when your patience occasionally runs thin.

The work of creating safety for your child during divorce doesn't happen in grand gestures or perfect moments. It unfolds in the quiet repetition of breakfast routines, the familiar rhythm of bedtime stories, the predictable way you say goodbye each morning and hello each afternoon.

These small, consistent patterns speak directly to your child's nervous system in a language more powerful than any words of reassurance you could offer.

When the ground beneath their feet has shifted, these routines become the solid places where they can stand.

You've learned in this chapter that predictability serves a biological function, not just an emotional one. Your child's developing brain relies on consistent patterns to determine safety, and when routines remain steady even as family structure changes, their body receives repeated messages that they can trust their world.

This matters profoundly for all children and becomes even more critical for neurodivergent children who depend on structure to manage sensory input, navigate transitions, and maintain emotional regulation.

The truth is that you cannot control what happens in the other household. You cannot force cooperation from an ex-partner who dismisses the importance of routines or whose own struggles make consistency impossible.

But you can create unwavering predictability in your own home, and that singular consistency provides your child with a secure base—a place where their nervous system can settle, where they know what to expect, and where they can count on you to show up the same steady way day after day.

Perhaps most importantly, you've discovered that repair matters more than perfection.

The moments when you lose patience, when your stress spills over, when your child witnesses conflict or returns from a difficult visit—these ruptures don't damage your child permanently.

What heals is your willingness to return, to acknowledge what happened, to reconnect with gentleness and take responsibility without burdening your child with adult explanations.

As Daniel Siegel explains, mistakes are a natural part of close relationships. This pattern of break and reconnection teaches your child that relationships can withstand difficulty, that emotions can be worked through, and that your love remains constant even during hard moments.

The cues your child sends when they need reassurance—the increased clinginess, the physical complaints, the repetitive play themes, the questions disguised as observations—these signals invite you to look beneath the surface and respond to worries they cannot name.

You don't need therapeutic training to offer what your child needs most: your presence, your validation, and your consistent reminder that they are safe and loved

Safety isn't built through elaborate interventions or expensive resources.

It's constructed through the accumulation of ordinary moments handled with care.

The way you maintain bedtime routines even when you're exhausted. The gentle repair you offer after a hard morning. The predictable rhythm of your days together that tells your child's body, again and again, that despite everything that has changed, you remain their steady place.

Your child doesn't need you to be perfect. They don't need two identical households or a cooperative co-parent.

They need you to show up consistently, to notice when they're struggling, and to reconnect when things go sideways. You're already doing this work, moment by moment, routine by routine, repair by repair.

And in these small, repeated acts of presence and consistency, you're building exactly what your child needs most: the unshakeable knowledge that they are held, that they matter, and that you will be there.

CHAPTER 6

When Behavior Is a Child's Way of Speaking

Understanding Changes in Play, Sleep, and Attachment

Your child's bedroom floor has become a recurring scene of chaos—the same dollhouse drama playing out night after night, where the mommy doll leaves and the baby doll cries, or where figures crash into each other with surprising force.

Meanwhile, the child who once slept peacefully through the night now appears at your bedside at 2 a.m., wide-eyed and anxious, asking to sleep in your bed, and mornings begin with a battle to separate for school that leaves you both exhausted and late.

These changes didn't happen overnight, but somewhere in the weeks since the separation, your child's behavior has shifted in ways that leave you worried and uncertain.

You find yourself asking whether this is normal, whether you should intervene, whether these are signs of something more serious—or whether this is simply how young children show what they cannot yet say.

The truth is that behavior is one of the primary languages of childhood, particularly for children ages three to eight who are still developing the vocabulary and emotional awareness to name complex feelings like grief, anxiety, betrayal, or confusion. You've seen this truth appearing intentionally again and again in this book.

Young children communicate through behavior.

When their world shifts in ways they cannot control or fully understand, children speak through their actions.

They show us their inner landscape through the stories they create in play, through their bodies' resistance to sleep or separation, through the ways they reach for us—or sometimes pull away.

This chapter explores three of the most common behavioral changes parents notice during and after divorce: shifts in play patterns, disruptions to sleep, and changes in how children seek or avoid connection with their caregivers.

Each of these areas offers a window into what your child may be processing internally, and each provides opportunities for you to respond with understanding and support rather than alarm or frustration.

Play is where young children work through experiences they don't yet have words for. Through repetitive scenarios, aggressive themes, or withdrawal from imaginative play altogether, children reveal what they're trying to make sense of.

Here's what I've learned from child development experts: play is both diagnostic and therapeutic—it shows us what children are struggling with while simultaneously helping them process difficult emotions in a safe, controlled way.

Sleep disturbances are among the most common and exhausting changes parents report during divorce.

Bedtime resistance, nightmares, frequent night waking, and requests to co-sleep often emerge or intensify during family transitions. These disruptions aren't manipulation or bad behavior—they're rooted in attachment needs and anxiety about separation, reflecting a child's fundamental question: "Will you still be here? Am I still safe?"

Changes in attachment behavior can be equally confusing. Some children become intensely clingy, unable to let their primary caregiver out of sight without distress. Others seem to emotionally distance themselves, becoming unusually independent or withdrawn.

Both responses are normal ways children attempt to manage perceived threats to their security, though they can leave parents feeling helpless or rejected.

For neurologically diverse children—those with autism, ADHD, sensory processing differences, or other developmental variations—these behavioral changes often appear more intensely or in less typical patterns.

A child who already struggled with transitions may experience profound dysregulation around bedtime or school drop-off. A child who uses play as a primary form of regulation may become rigid or repetitive in ways that concern caregivers.

Understanding these responses through both a developmental and neurologically diverse lens helps parents respond effectively rather than with worry that something is going terribly wrong.

This chapter will help you read your child's behavioral communication with greater clarity and confidence. You'll learn what different changes typically signal, how to respond in ways that provide comfort and security, and when shifts in behavior suggest a need for additional professional support.

Most importantly, you'll come to understand that these changes, while difficult to witness, are often your child's healthy attempt to process an enormous life transition—and that your consistent, attuned presence is exactly what they need to move through it.

What Play Reveals: Reading Your Child's Inner World Through Repetitive Scenarios, Aggressive Themes, and Withdrawal from Imaginative Play

When a child returns to the same play scenario day after day—staging the same family separation, crashing the same toy cars, or repeatedly making dolls "leave and come back"—parents often wonder whether this repetition signals something concerning or whether it's a normal part of processing.

What research has shown me is that repetitive play serves a critical function for young children working through difficult experiences they cannot yet articulate verbally. Through repetition, children attempt to master overwhelming emotions and events, transforming passive experiences of powerlessness into active scenarios where they control the outcome.

Tina Payne Bryson highlights that when children return again and again to difficult experiences, they are often working through feelings that are hard to put into words. In the early childhood years, emotional expression and understanding are still developing, so play becomes a safe and natural way for children to explore and slowly make sense of experiences such as parental separation.

Common repetitive scenarios include:

- Dolls or action figures repeatedly saying goodbye, leaving, or being separated into different houses
- Toy families being divided, with the child carefully sorting which figures "go with mommy" and which "go with daddy"
- Scenarios where a parent figure "forgets" to come back, doesn't show up, or falls asleep and won't wake up (particularly common when addiction is present)
- Reenactments of arguments, with figures yelling or being sent away

These patterns aren't cause for alarm in themselves—they're evidence that your child is actively working to make sense of their changed world.

The concern arises not from the repetition but from whether the child seems stuck in distressing loops without resolution, or whether the themes become increasingly dark without your child showing other signs of coping.

Aggressive play themes present differently but serve a similar processing function. When a previously gentle child suddenly begins crashing toys together with force, staging battles, or destroying block towers repeatedly, they may be expressing feelings they have no other outlet for—anger at the loss of their intact family, rage at powerlessness, or fear manifesting as aggression.

What the research shows is that aggressive play often emerges when children feel they cannot safely express negative emotions directly to us—either because they sense our fragility or because they've picked up messages that anger is unacceptable.

For neurologically diverse children, particularly those with autism or ADHD, aggressive play may also reflect sensory seeking behavior or difficulty with emotional regulation that's been intensified by the stress of family changes.

A child with ADHD may engage in more physically intense play as their nervous system seeks regulation through movement and impact.

A child with autism may show aggression in play when their need for predictability and routine has been fundamentally disrupted by the divorce.

The most concerning play change is often withdrawal—when a child who previously engaged in rich imaginative play suddenly stops creating stories, abandons their toys, or shifts to rigid, non-creative activities.

This withdrawal can signal emotional overwhelm, depression, or a child who has shut down their emotional world because it feels too dangerous or painful to explore even in play.

Child psychologists have helped me understand that this pattern can indicate a child's coping resources are depleted, particularly when combined with other signs of distress like sleep disruption, regression, or significant changes in eating or toileting.

Bruce Perry's work suggests that when imaginative play decreases, children may be experiencing higher levels of stress that make curiosity and creativity harder to access. When children are preoccupied with changes or emotional strain, playful exploration may temporarily give way to a stronger need for reassurance and stability. This pattern can appear in families experiencing conflict, inconsistent routines, or the unpredictability that often accompanies addiction.

What parents can do when noticing these play changes:

- Join your child's play without directing it, following their lead and providing gentle narration that helps them feel accompanied rather than alone with difficult feelings
- Avoid correcting or redirecting repetitive scenarios unless they're causing your child visible distress—allow the repetition to serve its processing function
- Provide language for feelings that emerge during play: "That little bear seems really sad that his mama had to go to a different house" or "The superhero looks angry—sometimes kids feel angry when big changes happen"

Sleep Disruptions as Communication: Understanding Bedtime Resistance, Nightmares, Night Waking, and Requests for Co-Sleeping Through an Attachment Lens

Sleep disruptions are among the most exhausting and emotionally charged behavioral changes parents encounter during divorce.

When a child who once settled peacefully into bed now fights sleep with tears and protests, or when a parent wakes multiple times each night to a frightened child standing beside the bed, the cumulative exhaustion can feel overwhelming.

These disruptions aren't random or manipulative—they're deeply rooted in attachment needs and represent a child's fundamental question about safety and connection during a time when their world feels uncertain.

Here's what I've come to understand about sleep from an attachment perspective: it requires a child to do something profoundly vulnerable — separate from their primary caregiver and enter a state of unconsciousness where they cannot monitor that caregiver's availability.

For young children, particularly those ages three to eight, this nightly separation depends on what attachment researchers call "felt security"—the internalized confidence that caregivers will remain available and responsive even when out of sight.

When divorce disrupts a child's sense of security, sleep becomes fraught with anxiety because it requires the very thing that feels most threatening: letting go of the parent they need to feel safe.

What the research confirms is that parental separation significantly impacts sleep quality, with studies documenting increased bedtime resistance, nightmares, and night waking in children experiencing divorce.

A longitudinal study of families found that parental relationship dissolution predicted poorer sleep quality at ages five and nine, with these sleep disruptions mediating later developmental and behavioral difficulties.

The study revealed that children's sleep problems following divorce weren't simply temporary adjustments but rather indicators of deeper emotional processing that required responsive parental support.

Bedtime resistance often emerges as a child's attempt to delay the separation that sleep requires.

A five-year-old who suddenly needs seventeen more stories, endless glasses of water, and repeated reassurances before bed isn't being difficult—they're communicating anxiety about whether their parent will still be there in the morning, whether the other parent is okay in a different house, or whether another loss might occur while they sleep.

This resistance intensifies when routines differ significantly between two homes or when children sense ongoing conflict between parents, as inconsistency erodes the predictability that allows children to relax into sleep.

Nightmares and night waking reflect the ways a child's nervous system processes stress during sleep.

When children experience high levels of anxiety or exposure to parental conflict, their hypothalamic-pituitary-adrenal axis—the body's stress response system—becomes dysregulated, leading to heightened arousal that manifests as nightmares or frequent waking.

Child development experts recognize these disruptions as the brain's attempt to process overwhelming emotions that the child cannot fully manage during waking hours. Dreams may feature themes of separation, loss, danger, or scenarios where the child searches for a missing parent—direct reflections of their daytime worries translated into nighttime imagery.

Requests for co-sleeping represent perhaps the most direct attachment-based response to divorce-related anxiety.

When a seven-year-old who has slept independently for years suddenly cannot fall asleep without a parent present, or when a four-year-old appears nightly at a parent's bedside asking to climb in, they're engaging in what attachment researchers call "proximity-seeking behavior"—attempting to restore sense of security through physical closeness with their primary attachment figure.

What the American Academy of Pediatrics has found is that sleep disorders, including bedtime refusals and nighttime waking, are particularly common among children who feel torn between two parents, two homes, and two different routines.

For neurologically diverse children, these sleep disruptions often appear more intensely.

A child with autism who relies heavily on routine for regulation may experience profound dysregulation when bedtime rituals differ between homes.

A child with ADHD may find their already-challenged sleep patterns further disrupted by the anxiety and emotional processing that divorce requires.

These children need even more consistency, patience, and understanding as their nervous systems work to find equilibrium amid significant change.

Changes in Attachment Behavior: Making Sense of Increased Clinginess, Separation Anxiety, and Unexpected Emotional Distance

What parents can do to support healthy sleep during divorce:

- Maintain consistent bedtime routines in your home even when you cannot control what happens at the other parent's house — predictability in one environment provides an anchor
- Respond to nighttime fears with calm reassurance rather than frustration, understanding that your child's nervous system needs to re-establish sense of security through repeated experiences of your availability
- Consider temporary co-sleeping arrangements if they help your child feel secure, while being clear with yourself about when and how you'll eventually transition back to independent sleep as your child's anxiety decreases

Attachment behavior—the ways children seek proximity to and connection with their primary caregivers—often shifts dramatically during divorce.

Some children become intensely clingy, unable to tolerate even brief separations from their primary parent. Others display unexpected emotional distance, seeming indifferent to comings and goings in ways that feel confusing or even hurtful.

Both responses represent normal adaptations to perceived threats to security, though they manifest in opposite directions.

Increased clinginess and separation anxiety emerge when children fear that the loss of their intact family signals potential loss of their remaining parent.

A four-year-old who previously separated easily for preschool may suddenly cling to a parent's leg, sobbing and begging them not to leave.

A six-year-old might follow their mother from room to room, unable to play independently even in their own home.

These behaviors reflect what attachment researchers call "proximity-seeking"—an intensified need to maintain physical and emotional closeness with the attachment figure to restore sense of security.

What research confirms is that parental separation correlates with heightened attachment insecurity in young children, particularly when family roles become unstable or when children witness ongoing conflict between parents.

Children in this age range often internalize divorce as personal rejection, developing beliefs that "relationships don't last" or "people I love leave me," which manifest as desperate attempts to prevent further abandonment through constant vigilance and physical closeness.

For children experiencing parental addiction alongside divorce, this clinginess intensifies.

Maternal substance abuse creates what researchers describe as "strong discontinuity of parental care," where repeated relapses, treatment episodes, or incarcerations erode a child's confidence that their parent will remain available.

Studies document that children of parents with substance use disorders show attachment disorder rates as high as 50%, with separation anxiety being a primary manifestation.

The unpredictability inherent in addiction—not knowing whether a parent will be present, sober, or emotionally available—leaves children in a chronic state of hypervigilance about their caregiver's whereabouts and condition.

Unexpected emotional distance presents differently but signals equally significant attachment disruption.

Some children respond to divorce by becoming unusually independent, showing little reaction when parents leave or return, appearing indifferent to transitions between homes. This pattern resembles what attachment theory identifies as "avoidant attachment"—a self-protective strategy where children learn to suppress their attachment needs because expressing them has proven unreliable or painful.

What child development experts have helped me understand is that this emotional withdrawal is a child's attempt to protect themselves from further hurt by preemptively disconnecting.

If a parent has become unpredictable due to addiction, mental health struggles, or simply the chaos of divorce, a child may unconsciously decide that caring less offers protection from disappointment.

Research on children in divorced families notes that some develop hyper-independence, prioritizing self-reliance when they cannot count on consistent caregiving across two households with different rules, routines, and levels of attentiveness.

In families affected by addiction, this emotional distance often accompanies what clinicians call "parentification"—a reversal where children take on caregiving roles for their struggling parent, suppressing their own needs to manage a parent's emotional or practical functioning.

These children may appear remarkably self-sufficient, but this independence masks profound vulnerability and unmet attachment needs that will likely surface in later relationships if not addressed.

Both clinginess and distance represent children's nonverbal communication about their internal experience of safety and trust.

Neither response indicates permanent damage, but both signal that a child's attachment system has been activated by perceived threat and requires responsive, consistent parenting to restore security.

Understanding these behaviors through an attachment lens helps parents respond with compassion rather than frustration, recognizing that a clingy child isn't being manipulative and a distant child isn't uncaring—both are simply trying to survive an experience that feels overwhelming to their developing nervous system.

When to Worry and When to Wait: Recognizing Normal Adjustment Responses Versus Signs That Your Child Needs Additional Professional Support

Watching your child struggle through the aftermath of divorce leaves most parents with a persistent, anxious question: Is this normal, or does my child need more help than I can provide?

The line between expected adjustment responses and signs of deeper distress can feel impossibly blurry, particularly when you're exhausted, worried, and second-guessing every parenting decision.

Understanding what constitutes typical processing versus concerning patterns helps parents respond appropriately rather than either dismissing genuine struggles or rushing to intervene when patience and consistency are what's truly needed.

Child development research has taught me that most children experience some degree of behavioral and emotional disruption following parental divorce, with symptoms typically peaking in the first three to six months before gradually improving as new routines stabilize and children internalize that their world, though changed, remains safe.

E. Mark Cummings highlights that shifts such as increased anxiety, clinginess, sleep difficulties, or stronger emotional responses are often part of how children adapt to stress. When these experiences gradually settle and children continue to participate in everyday childhood activities, they generally reflect adjustment and emotional processing rather than lasting distress.

Normal adjustment typically includes temporary regression in previously mastered skills—a five-year-old who occasionally wets the bed again, a seven-year-old who needs extra comfort at bedtime, a four-year-old whose language becomes slightly less sophisticated during periods of stress.

These regressions usually resolve within weeks to a few months when parents respond with patience rather than punishment, understanding that children often move backward developmentally before integrating forward progress during times of significant change.

Similarly, mood fluctuations are expected. A child may seem fine one day and tearful or irritable the next, particularly around transitions between homes or during moments that highlight family changes—holidays, school events where other children have both parents present, or bedtime when worries surface. These emotional ups and downs don't indicate pathology; they reflect a young child's limited capacity to process complex feelings consistently.

The picture shifts when symptoms persist beyond six months without improvement, intensify rather than gradually decrease, or begin to cluster across multiple domains simultaneously.

Research on children of divorce identifies several red flags that suggest a child's coping resources are overwhelmed and professional support is needed.

These include persistent sleep disturbances that don't respond to consistent routines and parental reassurance, particularly when accompanied by physical symptoms like frequent illness, chronic fatigue, or significant changes in appetite.

When a child's body begins showing signs of stress through repeated stomachaches, headaches, or a weakened immune system, their nervous system is signaling overwhelm that requires intervention beyond parental comfort alone.

Play that remains stuck in distressing themes without resolution beyond three to six months warrants concern, particularly when the child shows no other outlets for processing emotions or when play becomes increasingly dark, violent, or hopeless.

Children's play often evolves as they process emotional experiences, with early themes of conflict or separation gradually making space for repair, reassurance, and a stronger sense of safety. As Tina Payne Bryson explains, when this shift does not seem to emerge on its own, play therapy can provide a supportive environment where children receive gentle help in working through their feelings.

Attachment behaviors that don't respond to increased parental presence and consistency signal deeper insecurity requiring therapeutic intervention.

A child whose separation anxiety intensifies despite weeks of patient, predictable responses, or whose emotional distance hardens into persistent avoidance of connection, may be developing insecure attachment patterns that benefit from family therapy or child-focused intervention.

This is particularly critical for children experiencing parental addiction alongside divorce, as research documents that children of parents with substance use disorders show attachment disorder rates as high as fifty percent, with compounded risks for anxiety, depression, and later substance use themselves.

Additional warning signs include significant behavioral changes at school—sudden academic decline, social withdrawal, aggressive outbursts, or reports from teachers of concerning play or statements—and any indication of self-harm, persistent hopelessness, or references to wanting to disappear or not be alive, which require immediate professional evaluation regardless of the child's age.

Chapter Conclusion

The changes parents observe in their children's play, sleep, and attachment behavior during divorce are not signs of permanent damage or parenting failure—they are evidence that children are actively working to process an experience that has fundamentally altered their sense of safety and predictability.

When a four-year-old stages the same dollhouse separation scenario night after night, when a six-year-old appears at the bedside at 2 a.m. unable to sleep alone, when a seven-year-old clings desperately at school drop-off or withdraws into unexpected emotional distance, these behaviors represent communication from children who lack the vocabulary and cognitive development to express what they're feeling through words alone.

Understanding behavior as language transforms how parents respond to these difficult changes.

Rather than viewing clinginess as manipulation, sleep resistance as defiance, or repetitive play as concerning obsession, parents can recognize these patterns as their child's nonverbal way of asking critical questions: Am I still safe? Will you still be here? Can I trust that my world won't disappear while I sleep?

These questions deserve patient, consistent answers delivered not through explanations but through responsive presence—showing up night after night with reassurance, maintaining predictable routines even when exhausted, and allowing children the space to process through play without rushing them toward resolution.

Research confirms that most children experience temporary disruptions in behavior and emotional regulation following parental divorce, with symptoms typically peaking in the first three to six months before gradually improving as new routines stabilize and children internalize that their changed world remains fundamentally safe.

This timeline offers hope to parents in the thick of difficult nights and tearful mornings—what feels overwhelming and endless now will likely soften with time, patience, and the consistent message that the child's primary attachment figures remain available and responsive despite the family's restructuring.

The distinction between normal adjustment responses and signs that professional support is needed lies not in the presence of behavioral changes but in their intensity, duration, and trajectory.

Temporary regression, mood fluctuations, and increased need for reassurance represent expected processing when they remain mild to moderate and show gradual improvement over weeks to months.

Concern arises when symptoms persist beyond six months without improvement, intensify rather than decrease, cluster across multiple domains simultaneously, or begin to significantly impair a child's ability to engage in age-appropriate activities like school, play, and peer relationships.

Parents should trust their instincts when something feels persistently wrong, particularly when observing:

- Sleep disturbances that don't respond to consistent routines and parental reassurance, especially when accompanied by physical symptoms like chronic illness or significant appetite changes
- Play that remains stuck in distressing themes without movement toward resolution, or that becomes increasingly dark, violent, or hopeless beyond three to six months
- Attachment behaviors that intensify despite increased parental presence and consistency, or emotional distance that hardens into persistent avoidance of connection

For neurologically diverse children, these behavioral changes often appear more intensely or persist longer, requiring additional patience, specialized support, and understanding that their nervous systems may need more time and consistency to find equilibrium amid significant change.

Children with autism, ADHD, sensory processing differences, or other developmental variations aren't more fragile, but they do rely more heavily on predictability and routine for regulation—making the disruption of divorce particularly challenging to their systems.

The most important message for parents navigating these behavioral changes is this: your child's struggles are not evidence that you've failed them or that the divorce has irreparably harmed them.

These behaviors are evidence that your child is doing exactly what they need to do—processing, adjusting, and gradually integrating a new reality. Your role isn't to eliminate all distress or prevent all difficult feelings, but rather to remain present and responsive as your child moves through this transition, trusting that with time, consistency, and your steady presence, they will find their way back to security.

CHAPTER 7

Holding Space for Love and Disappointment

Visits, Absences, and Mixed Feelings About the Other Parent

Your daughter stands at the window for the third time in ten minutes, scanning the street for her father's car, her small body vibrating with anticipation and hope. When he's an hour late—then two—you watch her face shift from excitement to confusion to something that looks like grief, and you feel a rage and helplessness that takes your breath away.

You want to protect her from this disappointment, to somehow shield her from the reality that the person she loves so deeply can also be the source of such hurt.

Yet here you are, holding space for her tears while swallowing your own anger, searching for words that will comfort without making promises you can't keep or speaking truths that feel too harsh for her young heart to carry.

This scenario captures one of the most painful aspects of divorce for many parents—watching your child navigate the complicated reality of loving someone who disappoints them, who may be inconsistent, struggling, or simply unable to show up in the ways your child needs and deserves.

You may find yourself managing the aftermath of cancelled visits, soothing your child through transitions that leave them dysregulated and confused, or answering impossible questions about why Mommy didn't call on her birthday or why Daddy seems different during their time together.

The protective instinct in you wants to fix this, to make the other parent be reliable, to somehow erase your child's disappointment—but you cannot control another person's choices, and that powerlessness can feel unbearable.

What makes this even more complex is that children don't experience relationships in the either-or way adults sometimes do.

Your child doesn't stop loving their other parent because that parent is unreliable or struggling.

They don't weigh the evidence and decide to withdraw affection based on a pattern of letdowns. Instead, young children hold contradictory truths simultaneously—they can love their parent fiercely while also feeling hurt, angry, confused, or scared by that same parent's behavior.

They can long for time together while also dreading it.

They can defend their absent parent to others while privately grieving the relationship they wish they had.

Your role in this complicated emotional landscape isn't to make your child feel one way or another about their other parent, or to protect them from ever experiencing disappointment. Children are remarkably perceptive—they already know when something isn't right, when promises get broken, when a parent's presence feels unpredictable or unsafe.

Pretending otherwise or offering false reassurances doesn't shield them; it only teaches them not to trust their own perceptions or to believe they can't bring their real feelings to you.

Instead, this chapter will help you learn to hold space for the full range of your child's feelings about their other parent—the love and the disappointment, the longing and the anger, the hope and the grief.

You'll find language for validating their experiences without badmouthing or making excuses, strategies for preparing them for visits and supporting them through the aftermath, and guidance for what to do when a parent doesn't show up as promised.

We'll explore how to help your child understand that they can feel multiple things at once, that loving someone and feeling hurt by them aren't mutually exclusive, and that none of their feelings make them disloyal or bad.

This work requires tremendous strength and grace from you—to witness your child's pain without trying to eliminate it, to honor their relationship with their other parent even when you're furious at that person, to stay present and steady when everything in you wants to either rage or collapse.

You're not doing this perfectly, and you don't need to. You're simply showing up, again and again, helping your child navigate one of life's most difficult emotional realities: that people we love can disappoint us, and we can still love them anyway.

Preparing for Transitions: Helping Children Move Between Homes with Tools for Managing Anticipation, Anxiety, and the Emotional Weight of Goodbyes

Beyond the challenges of missed visits and disappointment, transitions between homes carry an emotional weight that adults sometimes underestimate.

For young children, these moments aren't simply logistical handoffs—they represent a repeated experience of leaving one parent to be with another, of saying goodbye when goodbyes already feel heavy, of managing anticipation and anxiety about what comes next.

Each transition asks something difficult of your child: to shift between two worlds, to carry their sense of security across physical distance, to hold their love for both parents even when moving between them feels confusing or hard.

Transitions are particularly challenging for children ages three to eight, who are still developing the cognitive capacity to understand time, the emotional regulation skills to manage separation anxiety, and the language to express what they're feeling.

Early childhood mental health research, including the work of Alicia Lieberman, highlights that young children may experience separations as emotionally challenging, even when they know the separation is temporary. This developmental reality invites caregivers to approach transitions with preparation, predictable rituals, and gentle support rather than expecting children to adjust quickly on their own.

Creating predictability around transitions helps children's nervous systems prepare for the shift. When children know what to expect—when the transition will happen, where it will occur, what the goodbye will look like—they can begin to build internal resources for managing the emotional experience.

A visual calendar that shows which days belong to which parent helps children ages five and up understand the rhythm of their schedule.

For younger children, simple language repeated consistently works better than complex explanations: "Tomorrow after breakfast, Daddy will come to pick you up. You'll have three sleeps at Daddy's house, then you'll come back here."

The ritual of goodbye itself matters more than many parents realize.

A brief, warm, consistent goodbye—a hug, a kiss, a specific phrase like "I love you and I'll see you soon"—provides an anchor point that children come to rely on.

This consistency communicates safety: the goodbye happens the same way each time, and each time the parent returns as promised.

Here's something that surprised me when I first learned it: prolonged or overly emotional goodbyes often increase rather than decrease children's distress, because they signal to the child that the separation is dangerous or that we lack confidence in their ability to manage it.

Anticipatory anxiety often shows up in the hours or days before a transition. Your child may become clingy, irritable, or withdrawn as the handoff approaches.

They may ask repeated questions about the schedule, resist getting ready, or suddenly develop complaints about the other parent's home.

These behaviors aren't manipulation—they're communication. Your child is telling you that the transition feels big and that they need help carrying the emotional weight of it.

Validating these feelings without trying to eliminate them helps children learn that difficult emotions are manageable.

Simple acknowledgment works: "I notice you seem worried about going to Mom's house tomorrow. It's okay to feel nervous about transitions. Lots of kids do."

This language normalizes the experience without suggesting the child should feel differently or that their anxiety means something is wrong.

For neurodivergent kids, transitions often require additional support.

Children with autism may benefit from visual schedules, social stories that walk through the transition step-by-step, and extra time to process the upcoming change.

Children with ADHD may need help organizing their belongings and remembering what to pack, along with movement breaks before the transition to help regulate their energy.

Highly sensitive children may need quiet time before and after transitions to manage the sensory and emotional intensity of shifting between homes.

The goodbye doesn't end when your child leaves. Many children benefit from a brief check-in call or video chat on the first evening at the other parent's home—not to interrupt their time there, but to reinforce that you remain connected even across distance.

When a Parent Doesn't Show Up: Supporting Your Child Through Broken Promises, Cancelled Visits, and Inconsistent Contact Without Blame or False Hope

While preparation helps with planned transitions, a different challenge emerges when the moment arrives and your child's other parent doesn't show up as promised.

Your child has been waiting, watching, hoping—and now you must help them make sense of an absence that feels, to them, like a rejection. This is one of the most difficult situations you'll face as a parent navigating divorce, because you cannot fix it, cannot undo the disappointment, and cannot make the other parent be reliable.

What you can do is help your child process the experience in ways that protect their sense of self-worth while acknowledging the reality of what happened.

When a cancellation happens, your child needs validation without false reassurance. Children often find comfort in adults who acknowledge disappointment with honesty and care. Alicia Lieberman's work emphasizes that children are deeply responsive to emotional authenticity. When reassurance does not quite match what children sense, they may feel confused, whereas gentle honesty can help them trust both the adult and their own emotional experience.

Simple, truthful language works best: "Dad wasn't able to come today like he planned. I can see how disappointed you are. It's really hard when someone we love doesn't show up." This validation acknowledges the child's experience without making excuses for the absent parent or offering promises about future reliability. It creates space for the child's feelings without asking them to carry adult explanations about why the parent didn't come.

Children will often internalize a parent's absence as evidence of their own unworthiness. Children ages three to eight tend to interpret events as revolving around themselves—what developmental psychologists call egocentric thinking—which means they often conclude that things happening around them are somehow about them.

When a parent cancels or doesn't show up, young children frequently conclude "I must have done something wrong" or "I'm not important enough." Your role is to explicitly counter this narrative: "This is not about you. You didn't do anything to make this happen. Sometimes grown-ups have trouble keeping their promises, but that doesn't mean you're not lovable or important."

Repeated cancellations require a shift in how you prepare your child for visits. Rather than building anticipation days in advance, consider waiting until the day of the visit to mention it, or even until the parent actually arrives.

This approach, recommended by family therapists working with high-conflict divorce situations, protects children from the cycle of hope and disappointment that erodes their sense of security.

You might say, "We'll see if Dad is able to visit today," rather than "Dad is definitely coming on Saturday."

After a missed visit, watch for behavioral changes that signal your child is struggling to process the experience. Increased clinginess, regression in previously mastered skills, sleep disturbances, or aggressive play themes often emerge in the days following a cancellation. These behaviors are communication — your child is showing you that they need extra support, reassurance, and connection.

Responding with patience and increased presence helps repair the sense of safety that the broken promise disrupted.

For neurodivergent kids, inconsistent contact can be particularly destabilizing.

Children with autism who rely heavily on predictability may experience significant distress when expected routines don't materialize. Children with ADHD may struggle with the emotional dysregulation that disappointment triggers.

These children benefit from concrete tools like visual schedules that can be adjusted when plans change, and from explicit coaching about managing disappointment: "When plans change and we feel disappointed, we can take deep breaths, talk about our feelings, or do something that helps our body feel calmer."

Throughout these difficult moments, your steady presence becomes the counterweight to the other parent's inconsistency. You cannot control whether the other parent shows up, but you can control how you help your child make meaning of the experience—with compassion, honesty, and the clear message that they are worthy of reliability even when they don't receive it.

After the Visit: What to Do When Your Child Returns Dysregulated, Upset, or With Confusing Reports—Reading Behavior and Responding With Care

When visits do happen, a different challenge often emerges.

Your child walks through the door after a visit with their other parent and within minutes the atmosphere shifts—they're crying over something small, throwing toys, refusing to follow simple requests, or clinging to you with an intensity that feels desperate.

Or perhaps they arrive with a confusing story: "Mommy said you're the reason we can't all live together," or "Daddy's friend was there and she was mean to me," leaving you uncertain what actually happened and how to respond.

These moments test every parent's capacity to stay calm and present, particularly when you're already carrying worry about what your child experiences during visits you cannot control or observe.

Post-visit dysregulation is one of the most common challenges parents report after separation, and it reflects the enormous emotional work transitions require of young children. Moving between homes activates children's attachment responses and requires them to shift between different environments, rules, expectations, and emotional atmospheres—often within a short timeframe.

This cognitive and emotional switching is genuinely exhausting for young children, whose brains are still developing the executive function skills needed to manage such complexity smoothly.

The dysregulation you observe isn't manipulation or evidence that visits are harmful—it's often simply the release of tension your child has been holding during the visit and transition.

When your child returns upset or behaviorally escalated, their nervous system is communicating that they need help returning to baseline.

Your first response should focus on co-regulation rather than conversation. This means offering your calm, grounded presence as an anchor—sitting nearby, speaking in a soft and steady voice, perhaps offering physical comfort if your child seeks it.

Here's what we know: young children regulate through connection with a calm caregiver—they cannot think clearly or communicate effectively until their nervous system settles.

Asking "What happened?" or "Why are you acting this way?" before your child has regulated often intensifies their distress rather than resolving it.

Creating a predictable re-entry routine helps children's bodies anticipate and prepare for the transition back. This might include a quiet snack at the kitchen table, time to play independently while you remain nearby, or a sensory activity like a warm bath that helps the body release stress.

The routine itself matters less than its consistency—when children know what to expect upon returning, they can begin to trust that this home will help them feel safe again even when they arrive feeling chaotic inside.

For neurodivergent kids, post-visit dysregulation often appears more intense and lasts longer.

Children with autism may need extended time in a low-stimulation environment to recover from the sensory and social demands of the visit and transition.

Children with ADHD may exhibit hyperactivity or impulsivitythat reflects their difficulty calming down after excitement or stress.

These children benefit from explicit sensory regulation tools—weighted blankets, noise-canceling headphones, movement breaks, or fidget objects—offered without judgment or pressure to "calm down now."

Confusing reports require a different kind of careful response. When your child shares something concerning, worrying, or that contradicts what you know to be true, the impulse to interrogate, correct, or react with visible alarm is powerful.

What research on children's memory and suggestibility has taught us is that young children's reports are highly influenced by the emotional reactions they receive.

When a parent responds with shock, anger, or intensive questioning, children often elaborate or modify their stories—not because they're lying, but because they're trying to make sense of the adult's reaction and provide the response they believe is expected.

Instead, receive your child's report with calm acknowledgment: "Thank you for telling me that. I'm glad you can talk to me about your visits."

Avoid immediate follow-up questions, corrections, or visible distress. If the report suggests potential safety concerns, document what your child said in their own words and consult with a family therapist or attorney about appropriate next steps but resist the urge to investigate through your child in the moment.

Holding Both Truths: Teaching Children That They Can Love a Parent and Feel Hurt by Them—Language for Validating Mixed Feelings Without Disloyalty or Shame

One of the most important emotional truths you can teach your child during divorce is that feelings don't cancel each other out.

A child can love their parent deeply and simultaneously feel angry at broken promises, scared by unpredictable behavior, or hurt by absences.

These emotions coexist, and holding space for both protects children from the corrosive belief that loving someone means accepting harm without complaint, or that feeling hurt means they must withdraw their love entirely.

Children maintain emotional bonds with parents even when those relationships involve disappointment or inconsistency.

What attachment research has taught us is profound: children are biologically wired to seek connection with caregivers regardless of the quality of care they receive—which explains why children continue loving parents who struggle with addiction, mental health challenges, or chronic unreliability.

This attachment persists not because children are confused about their parent's limitations, but because the drive for connection is fundamental to human development and survival.

The language you use to validate mixed feelings directly shapes whether your child experiences these emotions as normal or shameful. When a child says, "I hate Daddy" after a cancelled visit, the instinct to correct—"No you don't, you love Daddy"—is understandable but counterproductive.

This response teaches the child that their anger is unacceptable, that they must hide negative feelings to remain loyal, and that you cannot handle the full truth of their emotional experience.

Children need adults who can hold their most difficult feelings without flinching, collapsing, or rushing to fix the discomfort—this is one of the most important things we can offer them.

Instead, validation acknowledges the feeling while leaving room for its opposite: "You're really angry at Dad right now because he didn't come when he said he would. It's hard to feel excited to see someone and then disappointed when they don't show up. You can love him and be mad at him at the same time."

This language normalizes emotional complexity, teaches children that feelings are temporary states rather than permanent truths, and communicates that all of their emotions are welcome in your presence.

Children often need explicit permission to hold contradictory feelings without choosing between them. Young children in this age range struggle with understanding that two opposing things can be true simultaneously—it's a cognitive skill that's still developing.

They think in concrete, either-or terms: something is good or bad, safe or scary, loved or rejected. The concept that a parent can be both loving and hurtful, both wanted and disappointing, requires cognitive flexibility that is still emerging during these years.

You can support this developing capacity by naming both truths out loud: "I know you miss Mom and wish you could see her more. I also know that sometimes when you're with her, things happen that make you feel confused or upset. Both of those things are true, and both of your feelings make sense."

This explicit framing helps children understand that emotional ambivalence isn't a problem to solve but a reality to accept.

For neurodivergent children, processing mixed feelings often requires additional concrete support.

Children with autism may benefit from visual tools like emotion charts that show multiple feelings coexisting, or social stories that walk through scenarios where a character loves someone and feels hurt by them.

Children with ADHD may need help slowing down to identify and name feelings that shift rapidly, perhaps through body-based check-ins: "Where do you feel the love for Dad in your body? Where do you feel the anger?"

Throughout these conversations, your role isn't to defend the other parent, make excuses for their behavior, or convince your child to feel differently.

Your role is simply to witness and validate—to communicate through your steady presence that your child's emotional truth, in all its complexity, is safe with you.

Navigating your child's relationship with their other parent when that relationship involves disappointment, inconsistency, or absence is among the most emotionally demanding work you'll do as a parent through divorce.

You're asked to witness your child's pain without being able to prevent it, to honor a relationship you may feel angry about, and to hold space for feelings that shift and contradict each other moment to moment.

This work requires a particular kind of strength—not the strength of having all the answers or maintaining perfect composure, but the strength of showing up again and again to help your child make sense of experiences that don't make sense, to validate feelings that are messy and complicated, and to communicate through your steady presence that they are worthy of reliability even when they don't always receive it.

The research is clear that children benefit most when they can maintain connections with both parents whenever it is safe to do so, but this doesn't mean you must pretend disappointment doesn't exist or shield your child from the reality of who their other parent is.

Here's what I want you to know: children are remarkably perceptive—they already know when promises get broken, when a parent is unreliable, when something feels off during visits.

Your role isn't to create a false narrative that protects the other parent's image at the expense of your child's reality.

Instead, your role is to help your child understand their experiences with honesty and compassion, to validate their feelings without burdening them with adult anger or blame, and to teach them the profound truth that they can love someone and feel hurt by them simultaneously.

The language you use in these moments shapes how your child learns to understand relationships, disappointment, and their own worthiness. When you acknowledge that a parent didn't show up without making excuses, when you validate anger and sadness without requiring your child to choose one feeling over the other, when you explicitly counter the narrative that they are somehow responsible for another person's limitations—you are building your child's capacity for emotional complexity and self-worth that will serve them throughout their life.

You are teaching them that feelings don't have to be simple to be valid, that loving someone doesn't mean accepting harm without acknowledgment, and that they can trust their own perceptions even when the adults around them are struggling.

This work is exhausting, and there will be moments when you don't handle it perfectly—when your own anger slips through, when you're too tired to offer the patient validation your child needs, when the unfairness of it all makes you want to give up.

These moments don't undo the steady foundation you're building.

What matters most is your willingness to keep showing up, to repair when you stumble, and to remain the consistent, trustworthy presence your child can return to when their other parent cannot provide that stability.

You cannot control whether your child's other parent shows up reliably, keeps promises, or behaves in ways that honor your child's needs.

You cannot eliminate your child's disappointment or make their feelings less complicated.

What you can do—what you are already doing—is help your child navigate this difficult reality with their sense of self intact, their capacity for love preserved, and their understanding that they deserve better than inconsistency even when they experience it.

That is enough. You are enough. And your child, held in your steady presence through all of this complexity, will be okay.

CHAPTER 8

Protecting Your Child When Things Feel Uncertain

Boundaries, Safety, and Trusting Your Instincts

Something in your gut tells you that your child isn't safe during visits with their other parent, but you can't quite name what's wrong—maybe it's the way your son flinches when you mention Daddy's house, or how your daughter comes home smelling of cigarette smoke despite promises that no one smokes around her, or the concerning vagueness when you ask simple questions about their weekend.

You lie awake at night caught between fear for your child's wellbeing and worry that you're overreacting, that your own hurt about the divorce is clouding your judgment, that speaking up will make you look like the difficult ex trying to interfere with the other parent's time.

This internal conflict—the tension between protecting your child and questioning your own judgment—is one of the loneliest aspects of protective parenting during divorce.

You may feel caught between competing pressures: family court professionals who emphasize the importance of both parents in a child's life, your own desire not to be controlling or vindictive, and the primal instinct that something isn't right.

You might question yourself constantly— *Am I seeing problems that aren't there? Am I letting my anger at my ex affect my perception? What if I'm wrong?*

Here's what I've learned from the research on child development and trauma, and what I see again and again in my work: parents are usually the most attuned observers of their own children's wellbeing.

When you notice changes in your child's behavior, mood, or sense of safety that correlate with time spent with the other parent, those observations matter.

Children communicate distress through behavior long before they have words for what's wrong—and parents who pay attention to these signals are not being overprotective, they're being responsive.

This chapter is for parents who find themselves in the difficult position of needing to set boundaries or take protective action when circumstances with the other parent feel uncertain or unsafe.

Perhaps you're dealing with active addiction that hasn't been addressed, mental health concerns that affect parenting capacity, living conditions that worry you, or behavior that leaves your child anxious or dysregulated after visits.

Maybe you've tried to address concerns directly and been met with defensiveness, denial, or accusations that you're trying to keep the child away. Or perhaps the other parent seems fine on the surface, but your child's reactions tell a different story.

The goal of this chapter isn't to encourage conflict or alienation—quite the opposite.

It's to help you distinguish between normal divorce-associated anxiety and genuine safety concerns, to trust your observations while also examining them honestly, and to take appropriate protective steps when your child's wellbeing requires it.

You'll learn to read your child's behavioral signals more clearly, understand what healthy boundaries look like even in high-conflict situations, and navigate the practical realities of documentation and legal intervention when modifications to custody or visitation become necessary.

This work is exhausting and often isolating.

You may feel like you're fighting battles on multiple fronts—managing your child's distress, dealing with an uncooperative or hostile ex-partner, navigating systems that don't always respond quickly to concerns, and carrying the constant vigilance that comes with being the parent who's paying attention.

It's important to name this reality: protective parenting takes an enormous emotional toll, and you're not weak or failing if you feel overwhelmed by it.

Throughout this chapter, we'll focus on empowering you to trust your instincts, advocate effectively for your child, and take action when needed—even when that action is difficult or met with resistance.

Setting boundaries isn't about punishment or control. It's about creating the conditions your child needs to feel safe, and sometimes that means making hard decisions that prioritize their wellbeing over keeping the peace or maintaining an illusion of cooperative co-parenting that doesn't actually exist.

Trusting Your Instincts: Distinguishing Between Divorce-Related Anxiety and Legitimate Safety Concerns—When Your Gut Tells You Something Isn't Right

Understanding when your concerns reflect genuine danger versus your own anxiety is perhaps the most challenging aspect of safety-focused parenting.

The distinction between divorce-related anxiety and genuine safety concerns often feels impossibly blurry, particularly when parents are navigating their own emotional upheaval while trying to remain attuned to their children's needs.

Understanding this difference requires both self-awareness about one's own emotional state and careful observation of specific, concrete indicators in a child's behavior and circumstances.

Recognizing Divorce-Related Anxiety

Anxiety stemming from the divorce itself typically manifests in particular patterns. Parents may find themselves catastrophizing—imagining worst-case scenarios with minimal evidence to support them.

A child mentions that Daddy let them stay up late, and the parent's mind immediately jumps to complete neglect of bedtime routines, poor judgment, and potential harm. This pattern of thinking takes isolated incidents and expands them into sweeping narratives of danger.

Divorce-associated anxiety also tends to be generalized rather than specific. Parents experiencing this type of anxiety often worry about multiple aspects of the other parent's care simultaneously—the cleanliness of the home, the appropriateness of meals, the supervision provided, the emotional attunement offered. The anxiety feels pervasive and difficult to pin down to concrete concerns.

Another hallmark of anxiety-driven worry is rumination without resolution. Parents find themselves thinking in circles about potential problems, replaying scenarios in their minds, but unable to identify specific actions to take because the concerns remain vague and hypothetical.

Identifying Legitimate Safety Concerns

Legitimate safety concerns, by contrast, tend to be specific, observable, and documentable. Rather than a general sense of unease, parents can point to concrete incidents: a child returning home with unexplained bruises, a consistent pattern of the other parent driving while intoxicated, a child demonstrating age-inappropriate sexual knowledge, or living conditions that genuinely endanger health and safety.

What clinical psychologists who specialize in family trauma have taught me is that children communicate distress through behavioral changes that connect to specific experiences.

When legitimate safety issues exist, children often show clear indicators: regression in previously mastered skills, new fears that emerge specifically around transitions to the other parent's home, physical symptoms like stomachaches or headaches before visits, or explicit statements expressing fear or discomfort.

Legitimate concerns also tend to be validated by external observers.

Teachers notice changes in behavior following weekends with the other parent.

Pediatricians document injuries or signs of neglect.

Therapists observe trauma responses that align with the child's reports of experiences in the other home.

This external corroboration provides crucial perspective that helps distinguish between one parent's anxiety and genuine problems affecting the child.

Questions for Self-Assessment

Parents can develop greater clarity about their concerns by asking themselves specific questions.

Can the concern be described in concrete, behavioral terms? "My daughter comes home from visits smelling strongly of marijuana smoke" is specific and observable.

"I just have a bad feeling about what happens there" is not.

Have other trusted adults expressed similar concerns independently?

If a child's teacher, pediatrician, or therapist has noted worrying changes without prompting, that external validation carries significant weight.

Does the child show behavioral or emotional indicators that align with the concern? Children experiencing genuine harm typically demonstrate distress through their behavior, emotions, sleep patterns, or physical symptoms.

The absence of these indicators, while not definitive proof of safety, suggests that parental anxiety may be outpacing actual risk.

Is the concern about a safety issue or a parenting difference?

The other parent may have different rules about screen time, different standards of household organization, or different approaches to discipline.

These differences, while potentially frustrating, do not constitute safety concerns unless they genuinely endanger the child's physical or emotional wellbeing.

Finally, parents should consider whether they have a pattern of worry across multiple areas of life.

Generalized anxiety often accompanies divorce, and recognizing this pattern can help parents understand when their concerns reflect their own emotional state rather than objective threats to their child's safety.

Reading Your Child's Signals: Behavioral Cues That May Indicate Distress, Unsafe Conditions, or Concerning Experiences During Visits

Even when you've identified genuine safety concerns, understanding what your child is experiencing can be challenging.

Children ages three through eight rarely have the vocabulary or emotional awareness to articulate when something feels wrong during visits with their other parent.

Instead, they communicate through behavior—through changes in how they play, sleep, eat, and relate to the world around them. Learning to read these signals requires careful observation of patterns rather than isolated incidents and understanding that behavioral changes often intensify around transitions to and from the other parent's home.

Emotional and Behavioral Indicators

One of the most common signals that something may be concerning during visits is a marked change in emotional regulation.

Children who previously managed frustration with age-appropriate responses may suddenly exhibit intense emotional outbursts—screaming, hitting, or collapsing into inconsolable tears over minor disappointments.

Conversely, some children become unusually withdrawn, showing a flatness or emotional numbness that wasn't present before. These patterns of emotional regulation difficulties often reflect the child's attempt to manage overwhelming experiences they cannot yet process verbally.

Hypervigilance represents another significant behavioral cue.

Children who seem constantly on alert—scanning their environment, startling easily at sudden movements or sounds, or showing exaggerated concern about a parent's mood or whereabouts—may be replicating survival strategies learned in an unpredictable environment.

Hypervigilance in young children often indicates they've learned to monitor adult behavior closely because their safety has felt dependent on reading and responding to subtle shifts in a caregiver's state.

Physical and Somatic Responses

The body often speaks when words cannot.

Children may develop physical complaints that emerge specifically before or after visits—stomachaches, headaches, or vague feelings of being unwell that have no clear medical cause.

Sleep disturbances that correlate with the visitation schedule—nightmares, bedwetting after being dry for months, or intense resistance to bedtime on nights before transitions—can signal anxiety about what happens during time away.

Changes in eating patterns also warrant attention.

A child who returns from visits ravenous despite supposedly having eaten, or who hoards food in their room, may be experiencing neglect or food insecurity at the other home.

Conversely, loss of appetite or complaints of nausea around visit times can indicate anxiety about the experience.

Regression and Developmental Concerns

Regression in previously mastered skills often signals significant distress. A five-year-old who was fully toilet trained may begin having accidents again. A seven-year-old who read independently may suddenly refuse to try. An eight-year-old who dressed themselves may become helpless and dependent.

While some regression is normal during divorce adjustment, patterns that specifically intensify around visits or that persist for months deserve closer examination.

What research on children in families affected by parental substance abuse has shown us is that role reversal—where children take on adult responsibilities — creates distinct behavioral signatures.

Young children may return from visits describing having to wake up a parent, prepare their own meals, or manage household tasks far beyond their developmental capacity. They may exhibit a troubling maturity, speaking about adult concerns or demonstrating anxiety about the other parent's wellbeing that exceeds normal childhood worry.

Social and Relational Changes

Changes in how children relate to peers and trusted adults can indicate concerning experiences. Children who become unusually secretive, who avoid eye contact, or who seem fearful of disappointing adults may be carrying loyalty conflicts or explicit instructions not to share what happens during visits.

Conversely, children who suddenly become aggressive with peers, who violate others' boundaries, or who engage in age-inappropriate sexual play may be modeling behavior they've witnessed or experienced.

The key to reading these signals lies in pattern recognition rather than reacting to single incidents.

When multiple behavioral indicators cluster together, when changes correlate consistently with the visitation schedule, and when the intensity or duration of concerning behaviors exceeds what would be expected during normal divorce adjustment, parents have reason to trust their observations and take protective action.

Setting and Maintaining Boundaries: What Healthy Limits Look Like in High-Conflict or Unsafe Co-Parenting Situations — Practical Steps for Protection Without Alienation

Once you've identified concerning patterns in your child's behavior and validated your observations, the question becomes: what do you actually do about it?

Setting healthy boundaries in high-conflict or unsafe co-parenting situations requires a delicate balance—protecting children from harm while avoiding actions that could be perceived as parent alienation.

Boundaries in this context are not about control or punishment; they are about creating the conditions necessary for a child's safety and emotional wellbeing when cooperation with the other parent is limited or when legitimate concerns exist.

Understanding What Healthy Boundaries Look Like

Healthy boundaries in high-conflict parenting situations establish clear, enforceable limits that guide interactions between parents while minimizing opportunities for conflict to affect children.

Family law professionals and child development experts have taught me that effective boundaries share several characteristics: they're specific rather than vague, focused on observable behaviors rather than character judgments, and documented in ways that can be referenced and enforced.

In practice, this might mean establishing that all communication happens through a co-parenting app or email rather than text messages or phone calls that can escalate into arguments.

It might mean agreeing to exchange children at a neutral location like school or a public place rather than at each other's homes.

It might mean specifying exact pick-up and drop-off times and adhering to them consistently to provide predictability for children who struggle with transitions.

When safety concerns exist—whether due to active addiction, mental health instability, or other risk factors—boundaries become more protective.

These might include requiring that exchanges happen with a neutral third party present, requesting that visits occur in supervised settings until concerns are addressed, or establishing clear protocols for what happens if the other parent appears impaired at pick-up time.

Practical Steps for Implementation

The first step in setting boundaries is clarity about what specific behaviors or situations require limits.

Rather than a general feeling that "things aren't safe," parents benefit from identifying concrete concerns: the other parent drives while intoxicated, leaves children unsupervised with inappropriate caregivers, exposes children to domestic violence, or fails to provide basic necessities like food or medication.

Once concerns are identified, parents should document patterns rather than isolated incidents.

Keep a factual log that records dates, times, specific observations, and any corroborating evidence such as photographs, text messages, or reports from teachers or medical professionals.

This documentation serves multiple purposes—it helps parents themselves see patterns more clearly, provides evidence if legal intervention becomes necessary, and creates accountability.

Communication about boundaries should be clear, brief, and focused exclusively on the child's needs.

Effective boundary-setting communication avoids blame and focuses on specific requests tied to child wellbeing.

Instead of "You're irresponsible and I don't trust you," a boundary-setting communication might read: "For Emma's safety, I'm requesting that all pick-ups and drop-offs happen at the community center parking lot at the scheduled times. This will help her feel more secure during transitions."

Working Within Legal Frameworks

When informal boundary-setting doesn't work or when safety concerns are significant, legal intervention may become necessary.

This might involve requesting modifications to custody arrangements, asking the court to order supervised visitation, or seeking provisions that require the other parent to complete substance abuse treatment or parenting classes before unsupervised time resumes.

Here's what I've learned about family courts: they generally respond to specific, documented concerns rather than general allegations.

Parents seeking legal modifications should work with attorneys experienced in high-conflict custody cases and be prepared to provide concrete evidence of the concerns they're raising. Many jurisdictions offer resources such as court-appointed child advocate appointments or custody evaluations that can provide professional assessment of the situation.

Avoiding Alienation While Maintaining Protection

Here's the important distinction between protective boundaries and parental alienation: it lies in motivation and execution.

Protective boundaries focus on specific safety concerns and are implemented in ways that still allow for the child's relationship with both parents when safe to do so.

Alienation, by contrast, involves actively undermining the child's relationship with the other parent through disparagement, limiting contact without legitimate cause, or encouraging the child to reject that parent.

Parents can maintain this distinction by never speaking negatively about the other parent in front of children, supporting the child's positive feelings about both parents, and being willing to adjust boundaries when circumstances genuinely improve.

Taking Action When Necessary: Documenting Concerns, Seeking Professional Support, and Navigating Legal Intervention to Modify Custody or Visitation Arrangements

When informal boundary-setting proves insufficient or when safety concerns escalate, parents may need to take formal action to protect their children.

This process—documenting concerns, seeking professional guidance, and pursuing legal modifications—often feels overwhelming and adversarial, but it represents a necessary step when a child's wellbeing is genuinely at risk.

Understanding how to navigate this process effectively can make the difference between concerns that are heard and acted upon versus those that are dismissed or minimized.

The Foundation of Documentation

If there's one thing that serves as the cornerstone of any effort to modify custody and visitation arrangements, it's documentation.

Here's how family courts work: they make decisions based on evidence rather than allegations, and well-organized records transform your observations into verifiable patterns that professionals can evaluate objectively.

Family law experts have taught me that effective documentation focuses on facts rather than interpretations—recording what happened, when it happened, and who witnessed it, without emotional commentary or assumptions about motivation.

Parents should maintain a detailed, chronological log that includes dates and times of concerning incidents, specific descriptions of what was observed, and any corroborating evidence such as photographs, text messages, or reports from teachers or medical providers.

For example, rather than writing "Ex showed up drunk again," documentation should read: "March 15, 2024, 6:00 PM pick-up. Ex arrived with slurred speech, unsteady gait, and smell of alcohol. Neighbor Mrs. Johnson present and witnessed exchange. I declined to release child and documented refusal via text message."

Communication records deserve particular attention.

Save all text messages, emails, and communications through co-parenting apps that demonstrate patterns of concerning behavior—missed visits, erratic responses suggesting impairment, refusal to communicate about the child's medical or educational needs, or hostile exchanges that expose the child to conflict. These digital records create tamper-proof timelines that courts find particularly credible.

Parents should also document their child's responses to visits—behavioral changes, physical symptoms, or statements the child makes about experiences at the other home.

A parenting journal that tracks patterns such as "Every Sunday evening after returning from Dad's, Emma complains of stomachaches and has nightmares" provides valuable evidence of the child's distress, particularly when corroborated by observations from teachers, pediatricians, or therapists.

Seeking Professional Support

Before pursuing legal intervention, parents benefit from consulting professionals who can validate concerns and provide expert perspectives. A family law attorney experienced in high-conflict custody cases can review documentation, advise whether concerns meet legal thresholds for modification, and help parents understand what evidence courts in their jurisdiction find most compelling.

Mental health professionals play a crucial role as well. A child therapist can assess how visits are affecting the child's emotional wellbeing and may provide written reports or testimony about observed trauma responses, anxiety patterns, or developmental regression linked to time with the other parent.

For concerns related to addiction, substance abuse evaluators can conduct assessments that objectively document parental impairment and its impact on parenting capacity.

In some cases, requesting a guardian ad litem—a court-appointed advocate who investigates and represents the child's best interests—can provide an independent professional assessment that carries significant weight with judges.

These guardians conduct home visits, interview both parents and the child, and make recommendations based on their findings.

Navigating Legal Modification

To modify custody and visitation arrangements, parents must file a petition with the family court demonstrating that circumstances have changed significantly since the original order and that modification serves the child's best interests.

What courts generally require is clear evidence of harm or risk—active addiction affecting parenting, domestic violence, neglect, or other conditions that genuinely endanger your child's physical or emotional safety.

The legal process typically begins with mediation, where documentation often facilitates private resolution without prolonged litigation.

When court intervention becomes necessary, parents should be prepared to present organized evidence, witness testimony, and professional reports that establish patterns rather than isolated incidents.

Success in these proceedings depends on demonstrating specific, ongoing concerns tied directly to the child's welfare rather than general dissatisfaction with the other parent's choices or lifestyle.

Throughout this process, parents should remember that taking legal action to protect a child is not vindictive or controlling—it is an act of responsible parenting when circumstances demand it.

Trusting your instincts as a parent while navigating uncertainty about your child's safety represents one of the most emotionally demanding aspects of divorce.

The internal conflict between wanting to support your child's relationship with both parents and needing to protect them from genuine harm creates a burden that many parents carry in isolation, questioning themselves constantly while watching for signs that something isn't right.

This chapter has emphasized that parental instincts matter—that the observations parents make about their children's behavioral changes, emotional responses, and physical symptoms deserve attention rather than dismissal.

Research consistently shows that parents are typically the most attuned observers of their own children's wellbeing, and when patterns of distress correlate with specific experiences or environments, those patterns communicate important information about what a child is experiencing even when they lack words to express it directly.

The distinction between divorce-related anxiety and genuine safety concerns isn't always clear, and parents benefit from examining their observations honestly while also trusting the specificity and consistency of what they notice.

Concerns that can be described concretely, documented with evidence, validated by external observers, and tied to observable changes in a child's functioning deserve to be taken seriously and acted upon when necessary.

Reading children's behavioral signals requires careful attention to patterns rather than isolated incidents. When multiple indicators cluster together — emotional regulation difficulties, physical complaints, sleep disturbances, regression, hypervigilance, or changes in how children relate to others—and when these changes intensify around transitions to and from the other parent's home, parents have reason to trust their observations.

Young children communicate through behavior what they cannot yet articulate verbally, and learning to interpret these signals represents a crucial protective skill.

Setting healthy boundaries in high-conflict or unsafe situations protects children without crossing into alienation. Boundaries focus on specific, observable behaviors rather than character judgments, establish clear protocols that minimize conflict exposure, and remain flexible when circumstances genuinely improve.

The goal is never to eliminate a child's relationship with the other parent but rather to create conditions where that relationship can exist safely. When informal boundaries prove insufficient, legal intervention becomes a necessary tool for protection rather than a sign of failure or vindictiveness.

Taking action through documentation, professional consultation, and legal modification requires courage and persistence, particularly when parents face systems that move slowly or ex-partners who respond with hostility.

Yet this work—maintaining detailed records, seeking expert guidance, presenting evidence clearly to courts—represents responsible advocacy for children who depend on adults to recognize when they're not safe and to take steps to protect them.

Throughout this difficult work, parents should remember several essential truths.

First, setting boundaries and taking protective action is an act of love, not control.

Second, you don't need absolute certainty to trust your observations—patterns of concerning behavior and your child's distress are sufficient reasons to act.

Third, the exhaustion and isolation that come with protective parenting are real and valid, and seeking support for yourself while advocating for your child isn't selfish but necessary.

Your child's safety and emotional wellbeing take precedence over maintaining an appearance of cooperative co-parenting that doesn't reflect reality.

When circumstances require it, you have both the right and the responsibility to establish boundaries, document concerns, and pursue legal protections that serve your child's best interests. Trusting yourself in this work—even when it's hard, even when you're questioned, even when you feel alone—is exactly what your child needs from you.

CHAPTER 9

Caring for Yourself While Caring for Your Child

Strength, Softness, and Knowing You Don't Have to Do This Alone

You've been holding it together for months now—managing schedules, soothing your child's fears, navigating legal meetings and financial stress, showing up for bedtime routines even when you're so exhausted you could cry.

But lately you've noticed that the patience you once had feels threadbare, that small frustrations send you into tears or rage, that you're going through the motions of care while feeling hollowed out inside.

You're not failing—you're human, and you've been carrying an enormous weight largely on your own.

This chapter exists to tell you something you may desperately need to hear: taking care of yourself is not optional, and it's not selfish. It is, in fact, one of the most important things you can do for your child right now.

Here's what the research tells us: children regulate their emotions by co-regulating with their caregivers. They borrow calm from the adults around them when their own nervous systems are overwhelmed.

When you are chronically depleted, anxious, or running on fumes, your child senses that instability even when you're trying your hardest to hide it. They may become more emotionally dysregulated themselves—more clingy and prone to meltdowns—because the anchor they rely on feels unsteady.

This doesn't mean you need to be calm all the time or never show emotion. Rather, it means you need enough in your own tank to be present, to repair after hard moments, to respond rather than react. And right now, that tank may be dangerously close to empty.

Divorce can bring a quiet exhaustion that reaches beyond physical tiredness — the emotional strain of caring deeply for a child while managing uncertainty, conflict, and responsibility. Laura Markham describes this experience as compassion fatigue, a natural response to sustained caregiving without enough replenishment. Parents may notice feeling overwhelmed, emotionally stretched, or temporarily less able to access the patience and warmth they value, not because those qualities are absent, but because they are tired.

If this resonates with you, please know that recognizing your own depletion is not an admission of weakness—it's an act of honesty that allows you to make different choices moving forward.

This chapter will explore why your wellbeing directly impacts your child's sense of safety and security. You'll come to understand the connection between a parent's emotional regulation and their child's emotional stability.

We'll look at the specific signs that indicate you're running on empty—not to add more worry to your plate, but to help you recognize when intervention and support are needed.

You'll find practical, realistic self-care strategies that don't require hours of free time or abundant resources, because the truth is that most single parents navigating divorce don't have either.

These are small practices that fit into the margins of your day and actually make a difference in your capacity to stay present.

We'll also address one of the biggest barriers to self-care: the belief that asking for help means you're not strong enough or that taking time for yourself takes away from your child.

You'll learn how to identify and access support systems—therapy, support groups, trusted friends and family, community resources—and why building a network of support isn't a luxury but a necessity.

You don't have to do this alone. And taking care of yourself isn't taking away from your child—it's giving them the gift of a parent who has enough left to offer presence, patience, and love even on the hardest days.

Why Your Wellbeing Matters for Your Child: Understanding Parental Regulation as the Foundation for Children's Emotional Safety and Security

Children's nervous systems are not designed to regulate independently, particularly during times of stress and upheaval.

As noted earlier, co-regulation is a natural part of early childhood—children often find calm through the presence of trusted adults when their emotions feel overwhelming. Bruce Perry emphasizes that a consistent, soothing adult can help children feel safe enough to settle, offering the reassurance their nervous systems are still learning to create on their own.

During divorce, when a child's world has fundamentally changed and their sense of safety feels threatened, this need for parent's emotional regulation intensifies.

The child who once managed minor frustrations independently may now fall apart over small disappointments.

The child who slept peacefully may wake multiple times seeking reassurance.

These are not signs of weakness or manipulation—they are neurobiological responses to perceived threat, and the child's system is seeking the regulatory support it needs from the parent.

When a parent is chronically emotionally dysregulated—running on empty, overwhelmed by anxiety or grief, quick to anger or tears—the child's nervous system registers this instability. This happens even when the parent believes they're hiding it well.

Young children are extraordinarily attuned to their caregivers' emotional states, reading tone of voice, facial expressions, body tension, and energy levels with remarkable accuracy. A parent's attempt to mask distress while remaining internally chaotic sends confusing signals: the words say "everything is fine," but the nonverbal cues communicate danger.

When a child's experience does not match the emotional cues they sense from adults, they may feel confused or unsettled without fully understanding why. E. Mark Cummings' research highlights that children's emotional security grows from their confidence in their caregivers' ongoing presence and care. When parents are understandably tired or overwhelmed, children may respond with increased closeness or sensitivity as they look for reassurance that their needs will continue to be met.

The impact of parental dysregulation extends beyond the immediate moment.

Children who repeatedly experience their parent as emotionally unavailable or unpredictable begin to develop what attachment researchers call **insecure attachment patterns**—they may become anxiously clingy, constantly seeking reassurance that never quite satisfies, or they may become avoidant, shutting down emotionally to protect themselves from further disappointment.

These patterns, formed in early childhood, shape how children understand relationships and manage emotions throughout their lives.

Conversely, when parents prioritize their own emotional wellbeing — through therapy, support systems, adequate rest, and practices that restore equilibrium — they preserve their capacity to be the regulating presence their child desperately needs.

A parent who has processed their own grief can hold space for their child's sadness without becoming overwhelmed, just as one who has learned to manage anger toward an ex-partner can respond calmly when their child expresses love for that other parent.

Similarly, a parent who has built support systems and practiced self-compassion can tolerate their child's difficult behaviors without taking them personally or reacting punitively.

This is not about achieving perfect calm or never experiencing difficult emotions.

Children benefit from seeing their parents experience and manage the full range of human feelings in healthy ways. What matters is the parent's ability to remain fundamentally stable and available—to acknowledge their own emotions while maintaining appropriate boundaries, to repair after moments of disconnection, and to consistently communicate through words and actions that the child remains safe and loved regardless of what else is changing.

Parental regulation, then, is not a luxury or an abstract ideal. It is the foundation upon which children's emotional security rests during one of the most destabilizing experiences of their young lives.

Recognizing When You're Running on Empty: Signs of Burnout, Compassion Fatigue, and Chronic Stress—and Why Acknowledging Depletion Isn't Weakness

Depletion doesn't announce itself with a single dramatic moment but accumulates gradually, showing up in patterns that parents often dismiss as temporary stress or normal exhaustion.

Recognizing the specific signs of burnout, compassion fatigue, and chronic stress allows parents to intervene before reaching a crisis point—and understanding these signs as legitimate responses to overwhelming circumstances rather than personal failures is essential for seeking help.

Physical exhaustion is often the first noticeable indicator. Parents describe feeling tired in a way that sleep doesn't fix, experiencing a bone-deep fatigue that persists even after a full night's rest.

This may manifest as frequent headaches, muscle tension, digestive problems, or increased susceptibility to illness as the immune system weakens under prolonged stress.

The National Institutes of Health has identified chronic fatigue as a hallmark of parental burnout. This is particularly true among caregivers managing high-conflict situations or a co-parent's addiction.

Emotional detachment represents another critical warning sign.

Parents may notice they're going through the motions of care—preparing meals, managing bedtime, responding to questions—while feeling emotionally distant or numb.

At times, the warmth and ease that once shaped interactions with a child may feel harder to access, replaced by a sense of emotional distance or fatigue. Moïra Mikolajczak's research on caregiver burnout describes this experience as a form of emotional exhaustion connected to the parenting role — a temporary draining of the energy that supports presence, patience, and connection.

Irritability and shortened patience often intensify as depletion deepens.

Small frustrations that a parent would normally handle calmly—a spilled drink, a child's repeated question, minor sibling conflict—trigger disproportionate anger or tears.

Parents may find themselves snapping at their children over trivial matters, then feeling overwhelming guilt afterward, which further depletes emotional reserves in a painful cycle.

Cognitive symptoms include difficulty concentrating, memory problems, and decision fatigue. Parents describe feeling unable to think clearly, forgetting important appointments or tasks, or becoming paralyzed when facing even simple choices.

This cognitive fog reflects the brain's response to chronic stress—the prefrontal cortex, responsible for executive function and emotional regulation, becomes impaired when the nervous system remains in prolonged states of activation.

Loss of pleasure and motivation extends beyond parenting.

Activities that once brought joy—hobbies, time with friends, exercise—feel like burdens rather than sources of restoration.

Parents may isolate themselves socially, cancel plans repeatedly, or spend free moments scrolling mindlessly through screens rather than engaging in genuinely restorative activities.

Sleep disturbances create a vicious cycle of depletion.

Some parents struggle to fall asleep despite exhaustion, their minds racing with worries about their child's wellbeing, legal concerns, or financial stress.

Others sleep fitfully, waking frequently, or experience early morning waking accompanied by immediate anxiety.

Still others sleep excessively, using sleep as escape from overwhelming feelings.

Increased reliance on substances to manage stress represents a particularly concerning sign. Parents may notice they're drinking more alcohol to unwind at night, using cannabis more frequently, or depending on caffeine to function during the day.

Studies in the Journal of Family Psychology show that parental stress significantly increases risk for substance use disorders, particularly among parents navigating divorce from a partner with addiction issues.

Fantasies of escape signal severe depletion. These range from daydreams about running away or disappearing to more concerning thoughts about self-harm or suicide. Any thoughts of harming oneself or one's children require immediate professional intervention through a crisis helpline, therapist, or emergency services.

Acknowledging these signs isn't admitting defeat—it's demonstrating the self-awareness and courage needed to change course.

Parents who recognize depletion early and seek support through therapy, support groups, or trusted relationships preserve their capacity to remain present for their children during an extraordinarily difficult time.

The SAMHSA National Helpline (1-800-662-4357) provides free, confidential support 24/7 for parents experiencing mental health crises or substance use concerns.

Practical Self-Care That Fits Real Life: Small, Sustainable Practices for Managing Stress and Maintaining Presence When Time and Resources Are Limited

The reality of single parenting through divorce leaves little room for the self-care advice that dominates popular wellness culture—hour-long bubble baths, weekend retreats, elaborate morning routines.

When a parent is managing all household responsibilities, navigating legal proceedings, and serving as the primary emotional anchor for a struggling child, the suggestion to "take time for yourself" can feel like a cruel joke.

Yet sustainable self-care doesn't require abundance of time or money. It requires intentionality about small practices that genuinely restore capacity rather than add to an already overwhelming list of things a parent "should" be doing.

Stress research suggests that gentle, repeated moments of self-care can offer meaningful support, even when time and energy are limited. Kristin Neff's work on self-compassion reminds us that brief pauses of kindness toward ourselves can ease emotional strain and strengthen resilience over time. For parents moving through divorce, this might look like placing a hand on the heart and softly recognizing, *"This is hard. I'm doing the best I can right now."*

Micro-practices that fit into existing routines offer the most realistic path forward.

A parent can practice deep breathing during the three minutes it takes for morning coffee to brew—four counts in, hold for four, six counts out, repeated five times.

This simple pattern activates the parasympathetic nervous system, shifting the body from stress response to rest-and-digest mode.

Similarly, a parent waiting in the school pickup line can close their eyes and do a brief body scan, noticing tension in shoulders, jaw, or stomach and consciously releasing it.

These practices require no special equipment, no childcare arrangements, and no additional time carved from an already packed schedule.

Movement as regulation rather than exercise reframes physical activity in accessible terms. A parent doesn't need a gym membership or a full workout — the American Psychological Association has found that even ten minutes of walking reduces anxiety and improves mood.

This might mean walking around the block while a child rides their bike, doing gentle stretches during a television show the child is watching, or dancing to one favorite song in the kitchen while dinner cooks.

For neurodivergent children who benefit from co-regulation through movement, inviting them to join in simple yoga poses or a brief dance party serves dual purposes—helping both parent and child discharge stress while strengthening connection.

Nutrition and hydration as foundational support often get overlooked when parents are in survival mode, yet basic physical needs directly impact emotional regulation capacity.

Keeping easy, nourishing options available—pre-cut vegetables, hard-boiled eggs, nuts, fruit—makes it more likely a parent will eat something sustaining rather than running on caffeine and adrenaline.

Keeping a water bottle visible serves as a reminder to hydrate, which research shows improves cognitive function and mood stability.

Strategic use of children's screen time allows parents brief restoration without guilt. When a child is safely engaged with an age-appropriate show or game, a parent can use those twenty minutes not to accomplish more tasks but to genuinely rest—lying down with eyes closed, sitting outside in sunlight, listening to calming music, or calling a supportive friend.

Becky Kennedy reminds us that parents benefit from real moments of rest, not just brief breaks between responsibilities. These pauses help caregivers replenish the emotional energy that allows children to feel calm, supported, and safe in their presence.

Identifying one non-negotiable daily practice—whether five minutes of morning stillness, an evening gratitude reflection, or a brief check-in with a supportive friend—creates a minimum baseline of self-care that persists even during the hardest weeks.

This isn't about adding pressure but about recognizing that small, consistent practices compound over time, gradually rebuilding the depleted reserves that make presence possible.

Building Your Support System: Identifying and Accessing Help Through Therapy, Support Groups, Trusted Relationships, and Community Resources—and Giving Yourself Permission to Ask

No parent navigating divorce and its accompanying challenges should carry the weight alone, yet many do—held back by the belief that asking for help signals failure or that they should be strong enough to manage everything independently.

A strong network of support can make a meaningful difference for parents moving through stressful periods, offering reassurance, shared perspective, and emotional steadiness that children can also feel. Suniya Luthar's research underscores the protective role of authentic connection, reminding us that stress is easier to navigate when it is not carried alone.

Building a support system requires identifying different types of help that serve distinct but complementary functions.

Professional therapy provides specialized expertise and a confidential space to process grief, anger, trauma, and the specific challenges of co-parenting after separation.

Individual therapy allows parents to address their own emotional needs without burdening their children, while family therapy conducted with children present helps rebuild trust, improve communication patterns, and reassure children they are not responsible for family changes.

Studies in the Journal of Family Psychology show that family-based therapy approaches—those that address behavioral health challenges from a family perspective rather than solely as individual matters—significantly improve outcomes for all family members and increase long-term stability.

Support groups offer something fundamentally different from individual therapy: peer connection, practical coping strategies, and the profound relief of knowing others understand the specific challenges being faced. For parents navigating a co-parent's addiction, groups like Al-Anon, Nar-Anon, and Families Anonymous provide structured support based on shared experience.

For those seeking evidence-based approaches without spiritual components, SMART Recovery Family & Friends offers science-based strategies.

Divorce-specific support groups help parents and children adjust to family structure changes, often in combination with counseling.

Children's support groups are particularly valuable—interacting with peers experiencing similar situations helps children feel less alone and provides age-appropriate tools for processing change.

Beyond formal support, trusted personal relationships form the foundation of sustainable help. Identifying two to three people who listen without judgment, respect confidentiality, and can provide both emotional presence and practical assistance creates a safety net for the hardest moments. These might be friends, family members, faith community members, or other parents who understand the realities of single parenting through difficult circumstances. The key is selectivity—choosing people who genuinely support rather than those who minimize struggles, offer unsolicited advice, or create additional stress through their own needs or judgments.

Accessing these resources requires overcoming common barriers. The SAMHSA Helpline (1-800-662-4357) provides free, confidential referrals to treatment and support services twenty-four hours daily in English and Spanish. Insurance providers, primary care physicians, children's schools, and community mental health centers all offer pathways to finding appropriate therapists and support groups.

Many services now offer virtual participation, addressing transportation challenges, childcare scheduling conflicts, and geographic limitations while providing flexibility that fits the realities of single parenting.

The most significant barrier often isn't logistical but internal—the belief that asking for help indicates weakness or that self-care takes away from children. The opposite is true. When parents model help-seeking behavior, they teach children that vulnerability is acceptable and that reaching out represents strength rather than failure.

Children whose parents actively manage their own mental health and build support systems demonstrate better emotional regulation, increased resilience, greater willingness to seek help when needed, and reduced anxiety about being responsible for their parent's wellbeing.

A parent's self-care directly strengthens a child's sense of security—the foundation upon which all other healing rests.

The work of caring for a child through divorce while managing one's own grief, stress, and exhaustion is among the most demanding challenges a parent will face. This chapter has explored why that work cannot be sustained without deliberate attention to parental wellbeing—not as an optional luxury but as a fundamental requirement for providing the emotional safety and regulation children desperately need during family transition.

Here's what the research tells us clearly: children's capacity to feel secure during divorce depends directly on their parent's ability to remain emotionally available and regulated. When parents are chronically depleted, running on empty, or overwhelmed by their own dysregulation, children sense that instability even when parents believe they're successfully hiding their distress.

The child's nervous system, designed to co-regulate with caregivers, cannot find the steady anchor it needs when the parent's internal state communicates danger rather than safety.

This doesn't mean parents must achieve perfect calm or never experience difficult emotions—it means they need enough in their own reserves to be present, to repair after hard moments, and to respond rather than react when children's behaviors communicate distress.

Recognizing the signs of depletion—physical exhaustion that sleep doesn't fix, emotional detachment from activities and relationships that once brought joy, irritability that surfaces over minor frustrations, cognitive fog that impairs decision-making—allows parents to intervene before reaching crisis.

These symptoms are not character flaws or evidence of inadequacy. They are predictable responses to carrying an enormous weight largely alone and acknowledging them honestly represents strength rather than weakness.

Sustainable self-care for parents navigating divorce rarely resembles the idealized images promoted in wellness culture. It doesn't require hours of free time, abundant financial resources, or circumstances that allow for regular retreats from responsibility.

Instead, it lives in small, intentional practices woven into the margins of already-full days.

Five minutes of conscious breathing while coffee brews. A ten-minute walk around the block. Strategic use of children's screen time for genuine rest rather than more task completion. One daily non-negotiable practice that restores even a small measure of equilibrium.

What the research shows is that brief, regular interventions produce more sustainable benefits than occasional intensive efforts, making these micro-practices not just realistic but genuinely effective for parents whose lives leave little room for traditional self-care.

Perhaps most critically, this chapter has emphasized that no parent should navigate this transition alone.

Building a support system through professional therapy, peer support groups, trusted personal relationships, and community resources creates the network of care that makes sustainable parenting possible.

Individual therapy provides space to process grief and anger without burdening children. Support groups offer peer connection and the profound relief of being understood by others facing similar challenges. Trusted friends and family members provide both emotional presence and practical assistance during the hardest moments.

The barriers to seeking help are often internal rather than logistical—the belief that asking for support indicates failure, that self-care takes away from children, that strength means managing everything independently.

The opposite is true. When parents model help-seeking behavior and prioritize their own mental health, they teach children that vulnerability is acceptable and that reaching out represents courage. They also preserve their capacity to be the regulating presence their child's developing nervous system requires.

Taking care of yourself is not taking away from your child.

It is giving them the gift of a parent who has enough left to offer presence, patience, and love even on the hardest days.

You don't have to do this perfectly.

You don't have to do it alone.

And the strength required to acknowledge your own needs and seek support is the same strength that will carry both you and your child through this transition toward healing.

CONCLUSION

If you've made it to these final pages, I'm guessing you've been carrying questions that feel too heavy to hold alone—questions about whether you're doing enough, whether your child will be okay, whether the decisions you're making today will shape their tomorrow in ways you can't yet see.

You've been navigating one of the hardest transitions a family can face, and you've been doing it while trying to protect the small person who depends on you most. And through all of this, you may have been searching for the perfect words—the right way to explain everything to your child.

Here's the truth: there are no perfect words to say to your child about divorce.

There's no flawless way to co-parent with someone who may be struggling, uncooperative, or unsafe.

You will have hard days when your patience runs thin, when your child's big feelings overwhelm you both, when you wonder if you're making the right choices.

But here's what matters more than perfection: your willingness to show up, to notice, to repair, and to keep trying even when it's hard.

Your child doesn't need you to have all the answers.

They don't need you to be calm every single moment or to shield them from every difficult emotion.

What they need most is to feel safe with you.

They need to know that even when life changes, even when they're angry or scared or confused, you will still be there. They need to see that feelings can be big and still manageable at the same time.

Mistakes can be repaired and relationships can be mended. And love doesn't disappear when circumstances shift.

Throughout this book, you've encountered strategies for talking with your child honestly and kindly, for reading the behavior that serves as their language, and for creating safety through routine and presence.

You've also learned about protecting them when it's necessary while honoring their need to love both parents.

You've learned that children can hold contradictory feelings—love and disappointment, anger and attachment—and that your role isn't to fix those feelings but to help your child carry them without shame or confusion.

If your child's other parent is struggling with addiction or other serious issues, you've been given permission to trust your instincts and set boundaries that prioritize safety.

You've learned to speak truthfully in age-appropriate ways rather than maintaining silence that breeds fear.

You've learned that protecting your child sometimes means making decisions that feel lonely or are met with resistance.

This kind of advocacy is an act of profound love.

But advocacy alone isn't sustainable without self-care. You've also been reminded that you cannot pour from an empty cup.

Caring for yourself isn't selfish but essential. Asking for help isn't weakness but wisdom.

Your own regulation and wellbeing directly impact your child's sense of security. The strength you show your child isn't about never struggling; it's about continuing to show up even when you are struggling.

Your child is watching you navigate this transition. What they're learning goes beyond the specifics of divorce.

They're learning that hard things can be faced. Feelings can be named and survived.

People can make difficult choices out of love. Safety and connection can be rebuilt even after loss.

They're learning these things not because you're doing everything perfectly, but because you're doing it with intention, care, and commitment to their wellbeing—even when your own heart is heavy.

Even knowing this, the road ahead may still feel uncertain. There will be more hard conversations. More moments when you question yourself. More days when you wish things were different. But you are not alone in this, and your child is more resilient than you might fear—especially with you as their anchor.

You are enough. Your love is enough. And your child, held in that love, will find their way through this change and into whatever comes next. Keep going. Keep noticing. Keep showing up. That is what will carry you both forward.

GLOSSARY

Attachment: The deep emotional bond a child forms with the adults who care for them. Secure attachment grows when children feel safe, comforted, and understood—especially during difficult moments.

Behavioral Communication: The understanding that children often express needs, fear, confusion, or distress through behavior rather than words. What looks like misbehavior is often a child trying to communicate something important.

Co-regulation: The process of an adult helping a child calm their emotions and body through presence, tone, and connection. Children learn self-regulation by first experiencing co-regulation.

See also: Self-regulation, Dysregulation

Dysregulation: A state in which a child feels emotionally or physically overwhelmed and cannot easily calm themselves. Dysregulation is not intentional misbehavior — it is a sign the child's nervous system needs support and safety.

See also: Co-regulation, Nervous System Response

Emotional Safety: A child's sense that their feelings are accepted, their needs matter, and they will not be rejected or punished for expressing distress.

Executive Functioning: The mental skills that help children plan, focus, remember instructions, and manage impulses. These skills develop slowly and are often affected during times of stress or family change.

Masking: When a child hides feelings, confusion, or distress in order to appear "okay," avoid conflict, or protect relationships.

Nervous System Response: The body's automatic reaction to stress, fear, or uncertainty. Children may respond by becoming clingy, withdrawn, irritable, hyperactive, or unusually quiet.

Reassurance Seeking: Repeated questions or behaviors a child uses to confirm that they are safe, loved, and not at fault for changes happening around them.

Regression: A temporary return to earlier behaviors (bedwetting, clinginess, baby talk, sleep disruption) during times of stress. Regression is a sign of emotional overload, not failure.

Self-regulation: A child's growing ability to manage emotions, behavior, and physical responses. This skill develops gradually through supportive relationships.

See also: Co-regulation

Sensory Overload: When a child becomes overwhelmed by sounds, touch, activity, or emotional intensity, leading to irritability, shutdown, or strong reactions.

Stimming: Repetitive movements or sounds that help some children regulate their bodies, manage sensory input, or express emotion. For many children, stimming is calming and protective.

Transition Stress: Emotional difficulty surrounding changes in routine, environment, or caregivers. Even positive transitions can feel overwhelming for children.

Trauma Response: Emotional or behavioral reactions that occur when a child experiences fear, instability, or loss of predictability. Responses may include withdrawal, anger, clinginess, or anxiety.

These terms are not labels or diagnoses. They are gentle ways to understand what children may be experiencing beneath the surface. When we understand the language of children's behavior, we are better able to offer steadiness, comfort, and connection.

This book draws on established research and the work of clinicians in early childhood development, trauma, and family psychology. Sources that directly informed the material appear in Works Consulted, while additional authors are included in Further Reading for parents who wish to explore these ideas more deeply.

WORKS CONSULTED

Alcohol and Drug Foundation. (2025, June 2). *Explaining addiction to a child.* https://adf.org.au/talking-about-drugs/parenting-talk/children-preteens/explaining-addiction-child/

American Academy of Pediatrics. (2019, July 3). *Sleep problems after separation or divorce.* HealthyChildren.org. https://www.healthychildren.org/English/healthy-living/sleep/Pages/Sleep-Problems-After-Separation-or-Divorce.aspx

Bogdán, P. M., Varga, K., Tóth, L., Gróf, K., & Pakai, A. (2025, July 4). *Parental burnout: A progressive condition potentially compromising family well-being—A narrative review*. PubMed Central. https://pmc.ncbi.nlm.nih.gov/articles/PMC12249155/

Brosi, M., Montoya, B., & Masri, K. (2019, December). *Helping children of divorce understand their feelings*. Oklahoma State University Extension. https://extension.okstate.edu/fact-sheets/helping-children-of-divorce-understand-their-feelings.html

Bryson, T. P., & Siegel, D. J. (2011). *The whole-brain child.* Delacorte Press. Drug Free Kids Canada. (n.d.). Make your drug safety conversations appropriate to your child's age. https://www.drugfreekidscanada.org/talk/the-importance-of-communication/age-appropriate-conversations/

Gorski, R. (2025, March 8). *Navigating divorce with neurodivergent kids* Pt. 1 (S8E05). The Autism Dad. https://www.theautismdad.com/2025/03/08/navigating-divorce-with-neurodivergent-kids-pt-1-s8e05/

Greig, B., Giraud, R., & Rudkin, A. (2023). *Separating with children 101* (3rd ed.). Bath Publishing.

Partnership to End Addiction. (2023, September). *Prevention tips for every age.* https://drugfree.org/article/prevention-tips-for-every-age/

Pedro-Carroll, J. A. (2020, November). *How parents can help children cope with separation/divorce*. Encyclopedia on Early Childhood Development. https://www.child-encyclopedia.com/divorce-and-separation/according-experts/how-parents-can-help-children-cope-separationdivorce

Queensland Government. (2025, December 19). *Explaining alcohol and drug use*. Child Safety Practice Manual. https://cspm.csyw.qld.gov.au/practice-kits/alcohol-and-other-drugs/working-with-children/responding-1/explaining-aod-use

Rudd, B. N. (2018, November 17). *Parental relationship dissolution and child development: The role of child sleep quality.* PubMed Central. https://pmc.ncbi.nlm.nih.gov/articles/PMC6369723/

SAFE Project. (n.d.). *Lessons learned: Talking to young children about a loved one's substance use.* https://www.safeproject.us/resource/talking-to-young-children-about-a-loved-ones-substance-use/

Sesame Workshop. (n.d.). *Explaining addiction.* https://sesameworkshop.org/resources/explaining-addiction/

Strasheim, C. R., Durden, T. R., & Cruickshank, K. (2013). *How divorce affects children: Developmental stages.* University of Nebraska–Lincoln Extension. https://extensionpubs.unl.edu/publication/g2209/na/pdf/view

Substance Abuse and Mental Health Services Administration. (2023, June 9). *SAMHSA*'s National Helpline. https://www.samhsa.gov/find-help/helplines/national-helpline

Today's Parent. (2018, May 1). *How to tell kids about divorce: An age-by-age gui*de. https://www.todaysparent.com/family/kids-and-divorce-an-age-by-age-guide/

Triple P Parenting. (2024, October 4). *Apart but together: Co-parenting* after separation or divorce. https://www.triplep-parenting.com/us/articles-and-news/post/apart-but-together-co-parenting-after-separation-or-divorce/

FURTHER READING

These books offer additional guidance and perspective for parents seeking deeper understanding and support.

Herlem, F. C. (2008). *Great answers to difficult questions about divorce: What children need to know.* Jessica Kingsley Publishers.

Kennedy, B. (2022). *Good inside*. Harper Wave.

Landreth, G. L. (2012). *Play Therapy: The Art of the Relationship*. Routledge.

Lieberman, A. F., & Van Horn, P. (2008). *Psychotherapy with infants and young children.* Guilford Press.

Lippman, J. (2008). *Divorcing with children: Expert answers to tough questions from parents and children*. Praeger.

Luthar, S. (2015). *Resilience in Development*. Cambridge University Press.

Markham, L. (2012). *Peaceful Parent, Happy Kids*. Tarcher Perigee.

Mikolajczak, M., & Roskam, I. (2018). *Parental Burnout*. Springer.

Neff, K. (2011). *Self-compassion.* William Morrow.

Porges, S. (2011). *The polyvagal theory.* Norton.

Sanford, D. (1995). *How to answer tough questions kids ask*. Multnomah Books.

RESOURCES FOR PARENTS

If you or your child need additional support, the following organizations offer guidance, education, and connection for families navigating separation, substance use, and emotional challenges. Reaching out for support is an act of care—for both yourself and your child.

Emotional and Mental Health Support:

- *SAMHSA National Helpline*

A free, confidential service offering treatment referral and information for individuals and families facing mental health or substance use challenges. https://www.samhsa.gov/find-help/helplines/national-helpline

Substance Use and Family Support

- *Partnership to End Addiction*

Education, coaching, and practical resources for families affected by substance use. https://drugfree.org/

- *SAFE Project*

Support, prevention education, and recovery resources for individuals and families impacted by addiction. https://www.safeproject.us/

- *Alcohol and Drug Foundation (Parenting Resources)*

Guidance for discussing substance use with children in developmentally appropriate ways. https://adf.org.au/

Parenting and Child Development Guidance

- *HealthyChildren.org (American Academy of Pediatrics)*

Trusted developmental guidance on sleep, emotional health, and adjustment during family transitions. https://www.healthychildren.org/

- *Triple P Parenting*

Evidence-based parenting strategies that support children through stress, change, and emotional challenges. https://www.triplep-parenting.com/

Talking with Children About Difficult Topics

- *Sesame Workshop Resources*

Child-friendly materials designed to help families talk about addiction, emotions, and difficult experiences. https://sesameworkshop.org/resources/explaining-addiction.

You do not have to navigate this alone. Support, understanding, and compassionate guidance are available for both you and your child.

ABOUT THE AUTHOR

Laura Bennett, M.Ed.

Laura Bennett is an educator and writer who supports parents navigating family change with a focus on the emotional well-being of young children ages three to eight. A first-generation American raised in a middle-class family, her understanding of how deeply family instability affects children was shaped early—both through her own family history and through years of working closely with young learners and their families.

Laura holds a master's degree in education and spent several years working directly with small children in early learning environments. During that time, she listened to the lived experiences of children impacted by parental incarceration, foster care, abuse, trauma, learning differences, and divorce. Later, her work with children with autism, ADHD, dyslexia, and other learning needs deepened her awareness of how emotional stress and developmental differences often intersect—especially during periods of family transition.

Known for her empathic and observant approach, Laura writes with careful attention to what young children feel but may not yet be able to say. Her guidance helps parents recognize emotional signals expressed through behavior, play, routine disruption, and regulation challenges, and respond in ways that foster safety, trust, and resilience.

Her work focuses on helping parents protect children's emotional safety during family change.

MORE FROM THE STEADY GROUND SERIES

The *Steady Ground Series* is designed to support parents and young children through life's most tender and uncertain transitions. Each book offers calm guidance, developmentally sensitive language, and reassurance that emotional security can remain steady even when family circumstances change.

If this book has been helpful to you, other titles in the series may offer additional comfort, understanding, and practical support as your family continues to grow and adapt.

Available titles

Talking to Young Children Ages 3–8 About Divorce and Parental Addiction: Answering the Hard Questions with Compassion and Clarity

A compassionate guide to helping young children understand family change while preserving emotional safety and trust.

Helping Young Children Ages 3–8 Navigate Life Between Two Homes: Answering the Hard Questions with Compassion and Clarity

A gentle guide to helping young children build stability, trust, and emotional security while living between two homes.

www.ingramcontent.com/pod-product-compliance
Lightning Source LLC
LaVergne TN
LVHW010355160826
845677LV00005BA/1286

9798999278821